THE WINE AND CHOCOLATE WORKOUT

Sip, Savor, and Strengthen for a Healthier Life

Greta Boris

Website: www.gretaboris.com

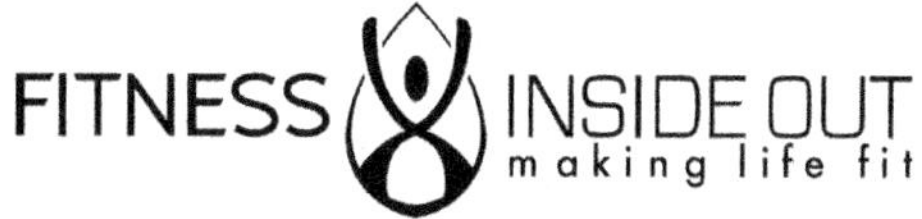

www.TheWineAndChocolateWorkout.com

Stop by www.GretaBoris.com and download free work pages for The Wine and Chocolate Workout.

Library of Congress Cataloging-in-Publication Data is available upon request

Edited by: Richard V. Howard

Jacket design by: Jake Melham Design
www.jake-melham.squarespace.com

Print and Electronic Editions Type and Format Design by:
Shawn E. Bell, www.shawnebell.com

v2.00

ISBN: 0692323732
ISBN-13: 978-0692323731

DEDICATION

This book is dedicated to my father and to my husband; the two greatest influences in my life. My Dad is my mentor, coach, and biggest cheerleader. My husband treats me like a princess, even when I act like the evil stepsister. He loves me, even when I'm unlovely. He supports my ideas, even though he doesn't like wine or chocolate.

Table of Contents

Acknowledgments

How many ways can I thank Jake Melham, my graphic artist? I love my cover art and his willingness to help me try to figure out the technical difficulties. Thanks to my "creative director," Kathy Bridges, who ran many miles with me discussing all the ideas herein. Thank you to Alison Stripling, my one-time business partner, for her great marketing ideas. And thanks to my new buddy, Shawn Bell, for his publishing wisdom.

Why Wine and Chocolate?

I WAS TRYING TO EXPLAIN TO MY HUSBAND what I was clicking away at the keyboard about for the past year. "It's not a diet," I said. "It's a book about how to change your waistline by changing your life. I want people to know they don't have to deprive themselves, give up everything they love to eat, or do boring workouts in windowless rooms."

"That's way too long for a title," he answered.

"I don't know how to express it in just a few words so people will know what I'm talking about."

My genius of a husband then asked, "What are two things most women you know would least like to give up?"

Without hesitation I replied, "wine and chocolate."

That's how *The Wine and Chocolate Workout* was born. Wine and chocolate are symbolic in my life for fun, joy, and healthy indulgence. Since I've had my children I have experimented with different ways to eat and exercise in order to "keep my figure" (as my mom used to say). Some were more successful than others.

The two guilty pleasures I have never been able to sacrifice on the altar of the skinny jeans, however, are wine and chocolate. I have gone gluten free, white sugar, white flour, white rice and white pasta free, dairy free (well, almost), stopped eating processed foods, have given up Diet Coke (that was rough) and even played around with being a vegetarian. But wine and chocolate—never.

During the time I worked with clients, I learned we all have our sacred cows. For some it's macaroni and cheese, for others ice cream. Some just aren't going to give up pizza and beer.

When we try to force ourselves into a cookie cutter (no pun intended) weight reduction program that takes away all our favorite treats and, even worse, bores us to death with counting calories, treadmill workouts, and food resembling roof shingles, how could we expect it to last? Over 90% of people who lose weight on this kind of regimen regain all their weight (plus change) within a two year period. Einstein defined insanity as doing the same thing over and over and expecting a different result.

This book is about turning forbidden foods into fuel, thinking deeply about a seemingly shallow subject like weight loss, and growing strong through our weaknesses. There are three things needed to change your life and your waistline: moderation, meditation, and acceleration. Real food isn't bad. It's just some foods have to be eaten in moderation, like wine and chocolate. Your meditations about yourself and your life are more critical to reaching your goals than how much wine and chocolate you ingest. You have to get up off the couch and move to reach your dreams. Wine and chocolate can provide the energy you need for that acceleration. So, you see, wine and chocolate, far from being forbidden fruit, can actually be critical to your success. You just have to get the right perspective.

How To Use This Book

One very effective approach trainers and coaches use to get their athletes ready for an event is called *periodization*. Periodization helps to prevent boredom, overuse injuries, and plateaus by constantly changing the type of work, the workload, and by building in periods of rest. It is based on the premise we don't progress in a straight line, but in cycles. In *The Wine and Chocolate Workout* we will be building in a periodization model with a healthy lifestyle change as our goal or our big event. Here's how it works:

1 Macrocycle - four months to a healthy lifestyle change

- **4 Mesocyles - one month each**
  - **12 Microcycles - one week each, with one week of rest every three weeks.**

Each mesocycle is developed with a different principle in mind, but each principal layers one on top of the other to help you reach your ultimate goal: the lifestyle change. It's the old how do you eat an elephant question. One bite at a time. If you break up the process into smaller steps, it will give you a chance to adapt rather than get overwhelmed.

These cycles are four weeks in length, three with action steps, and one week off to kick up your heels or ponder your navel. Experts say it takes about three weeks to create a habit, so you will practice new action steps for three weeks. Hopefully, by then these steps will no longer be an effort and you will be ready for the next set of action steps.

The microcycles are one week each. They are divided into motivational (mindset) topics, acceleration (exercise) topics and moderation (nutritional) topics. Each has a common theme. For instance, all the weeks in the first mesocycle are devoted to laying a foundation. If you look at the table of contents, you will see the outline of your training program.

As with any training program, you may feel you are already past the first section and may want to jump in on the second or third. I strongly suggest you read the preceding chapters anyway. Skipping steps that seem unimportant can trip you up later on. For a long time I resisted getting artificial sweeteners out of my life. When I finally did, it lessened my cravings for sweets, and that had a domino effect on my overall eating habits.

Here's my suggestion for making this program work. Use this book as a journal, or if you're reading the ebook, download the workpages at www.gretaboris.com. You will need to record your exercise, nutrition, thoughts and so on. Then each month:

1. Read the Mesocycle page and put it into action for one month

2. On weeks one through three, read one chapter each week and do the Meditate On It page

3. On week four, take a break.

Please take off the suggested time. It doesn't mean you have to stop exercising completely, or gorge on ice cream sundaes. Take a week off from thinking too much about all the changes you're making. Take time to treat yourself a little and relax your new disciplines. If you don't, you are destined for burnout. Remember, *this is for the rest of your life*. This isn't a *diet* you get to stop once you reach a certain predetermined weight on the scale. The breaks are designed to help you settle down with your new habits, make them your own, and make room for the next series of positive changes.

Mesocycle One
Shedding Fat Perspectives

During the next three weeks your goal is to assess your current situation. In order to get where you want to go, you have to have a good grasp on where you are. If you were my client, I'd run you through a battery of questionnaires, spend time understanding your current habits, and get to know what makes you tick. Following are some tools I've found helpful for gaining objective insight into client's lives.

Health Screening

First and foremost, this book assumes your health is good enough to embark on this lifestyle change without endangering yourself in any way. If you have any doubts, go have a physical. While you're there show your doctor the table of contents and ask if he or she has any hesitations or suggestions for you. Get some blood work or lab tests done. It is interesting to get as many objective measurements as you can. It can be very motivating to see cholesterol levels drop or other health markers improve.

Meditation Exercise - Objective Measures

Find a pair of jeans that are too tight, but you would like to fit into. Then close your eyes and vividly imagine fitting comfortably in those jeans. What does it feel like to zip them up easily; to bend over or squat to pick something up without having them pinch or pull; to look in the mirror and like what you see? Revive this picture in your mind every day. If you have an old photograph of yourself looking great in these jeans, put it where you can look at it daily. If you can't imagine it, you'll never get there.

You can also use the scale as a measure, but remember fat is light; muscle and water are heavy. If you only have a few pounds to lose and you're just starting an exercise regimen, the scale may not be the best indicator of the changes in your body.

Journal Work:

Record the following measurements in your journal and don't look at them again until next month:

Chest: ______________ Waist: ______________

Hips: ______________ Thighs: ______________

Weight: ______________

Moderation Exercise - Start Recording

Keep a food and exercise diary for the next three weeks. If you went to a financial planner and did not present them with accurate accounting records it would be very difficult for them to help you. It's the same thing with a food and activity diary.

You don't have to live this way forever, but you need a real picture of what is going on. I can't tell you how many clients I've worked with who've told me they eat "really healthy." They can't understand why they are continuing to gain weight. After doing a food diary for a month, they would see the ways in which they were sabotaging themselves.

There are several smart phone applications and free websites to assist you in this process. Check out:

- Lose it
- Fooducate
- Sparks People

These programs ask for basic statistics then let you know how many calories you need to maintain or to lose weight. It is almost universally true, people think they are eating fewer calories than they are. You have to face the truth to change the facts. If you are trying to lose weight, don't aim for more than one to two pounds a week.

Acceleration Exercise - Find Out

A helpful tool to give you a handle on how much you are, or are not, moving is a pedometer. They are relatively inexpensive and will record how many steps you take in a day. A study was recently done within an Amish community[1]. The Amish, by the way, have an obesity rate of 4%, compared with 30.9% for the rest of the country. The men walked, on average, 18,000 steps and the women 14,000 per day. Most Americans find it difficult to get to 10,000 steps.

[1] Bassett D.R., Schneider P.L., Huntington G.E. "*Physical Activity in an Old Order Amish Community.*" *Medicine and Science in Sports and Exercise. Aug;* 36(8):1447. 2004

Journal Work:

Sunday	Monday	Tuesday	Wednesday	Thursday	Friday	Saturday

Aim for at least 10,000 steps a day. Record those steps, or other exercise, in the calendar above or in a journal for the next three weeks.

ONE
Training Versus Trying

Recently, I was watching the LA marathon on TV. I know a little about running and I know how difficult and painful 26.2 miles can be. I found it amazing so many people of different ages, stages, shapes, and sizes had the determination to complete such a grueling event. What was propelling them toward the finish line? How did they accomplish this kind of life-altering goal?

After pondering this from my own experience of running races, I came up with three elements I believe are crucial: coaches, cheering crowds, and training.

Coaching

Coaching may come from an individual, a club or an Internet download. If these people ran 26.2 miles, they had some form of coaching. Any life-altering accomplishment comes with a thought-out, cohesive, educated plan. This book represents a training schedule designed to take you through the lifestyle changes necessary for success in the area of health and fitness.

Everyone's success will look different. Some people finished the LA marathon in under three hours, others took five. Their training schedules had to take into account the vast differences in their fitness levels, health, goals, and lifestyles.

Crowds

The crowds may not be necessary for everyone; some people are Lone Ranger types. However, most people are driven on the last ten miles or so by the encouragement of others. I was once injured part-way through a half-marathon. The last three and a half miles were so painful the only thing that kept me going was knowing my husband and friends were waiting at the finish line. Having a small group of friends who understand and are supportive, or better yet, who are attempting to make a life altering change themselves, can make the difference between finishing the race and giving up.

Whenever you attempt a big change you will find many nay-sayers. Sometimes they're in your family. Sometimes they're at work. Sometimes they come from your own head. You need positive voices to counterbalance the negative ones that will certainly come when the going gets rough.

Training

The last, and probably most important ingredient, is training. John Ortberg in his book *The Life You've Always Wanted*[1] talks about the difference between training and trying. He also uses the analogy of running a marathon. He states this seemingly obvious truth, even if you try really, really hard you won't be able to run a marathon without training for it.

---

[1] Ortberg, John. *The Life You've Always Wanted.* Grand Rapids: Zondervan, 2002.

This is true for most things that matter in life, from playing a musical instrument to running a business. There is always training involved when you begin a new venture. Why is it people think when attempting to change something as radical as how they eat, exercise, and look at life, they can do it by just trying really, really hard? Let's stop *trying* to get in shape and *train* instead. The following principles are the bones of this particular life-changing training schedule.

Training means making small changes with consistency and allowing yourself to physically and mentally adapt before another change is introduced.

Training employs small steps to reach audacious goals. There is a story told about Hercules. A heifer had a bull calf, and every day Hercules would pick up the calf and carry him around the paddock. He did this day after day, month after month, year after year. Eventually Hercules was carrying a couple of tons worth of bull around on his shoulders. Of course this story is bull, but it illustrates the point. Strength in every area is gained through small consistent steps.

Training will actually alter the physical makeup of your body, change your emotional state, and give you knowledge you can't unlearn.

When you swim, your body begins to build more muscle fibers in the muscles you use. It increases the number of oxygen receptors so those muscles become better at making fuel. Your heart grows stronger, and your lung capacity increases. You become a new creature over time. Every kind of training creates some kind of adaptation. We aren't stagnant beings.

We also adapt mentally and emotionally as we move through training. Think of the insecurity you feel when beginning a new job. Over time you learn what is required of you and gain the expertise to accomplish those requirements. The insecurity is then replaced by a sense of confidence.

Once you complete a training, you will always know the way to that particular finish line. I may not be in 10K racing condition at all times, but I know how to get there when I want to. The finish line in this training is the beginning of a new lifestyle. If you slip back into bad habits, you will always know the way out.

Training disciplines your body, working with it to bring out your natural strengths and abilities; it is not about punishment.

Many people fail in their attempts to get in shape. One reason is they indulge then push and punish to compensate for it. This is akin to bad parenting.

Have you ever noticed how the parents of a spoiled child discipline? Usually these parents give their child anything he or she demands, whether it's good for them or not. They confuse love with appeasement. This teaches the child to win their battles through temper tantrums.

At times, the parents have moments of clarity during which they realize they've created a monster. Then they decide to become super-disciplinarians. They are going to get their child whipped into shape. This, of course, never works because changing a child's heart and behavior takes years of steady, loving, discipline peppered with appropriate rewards and praise—in other words, training.

Think of your logical self as the parent and your body as

the child. Many people have spoiled their body, allowing it to run roughshod over their better judgment. Either they don't know how to discipline correctly, or they are terrified of the temper tantrums.

Whatever the reason you have allowed your inner-spoiled child to rule the roost, this book will give you the parenting skills you need to take charge. The only hitch is, you have to commit to applying what you learn even in the face of temper tantrums.

Meditate On It

Everybody has a belief system underlying their thoughts and actions. These beliefs may be true and accurate, or they may be faulty. Either way, they impact everything you do in life. I'd like you to do some soul searching and write down any beliefs, true or untrue, that may have frustrated your attempts to be lean and healthy in the past.

I went through a chubby phase between the ages of 8 and 11. I remember having a ballet teacher make fun of me in front of the class. Years later, even when I was dancing three hours a day and thin as a rail, I still believed, deep down, I was chubby and could never be as good as the thin girls.

Often these faulty beliefs become self-fulfilling prophecies. This page may be one you want to return to again and again. I've found the farther along people are in taking charge of their fitness, the more their eyes are opened to the things that held them back in the past.

Journal Work:

Record at least three reasons you believe you've been unsuccessful in the area of weight management or fitness in the past.

1. ______________________________________

____

____

2. ______________________________________

____

____

3. ______________________________________

____

____

- Now go back and analyze each statement for its truthfulness. Draw a line through anything you wrote that is not actually factual. For example, if you said, "I've always been fat, therefore I'll always be fat." Rethink that. You may have *always been* fat, but you don't have to stay that way.
- Next, analyze for defeatist thinking. Defeatist thinking says, "I can't change. The forces against me are too great." Turn around any defeatist statements and make them positive. For example, if you said, "I don't have the self-control to be thin." Re-write that as, "If I had the self-control, I could be thin." Now you know what to work on.
- Finally, look at the physical problems you are dealing with. "My knees, back, asthma, etc., are preventing me from exercising." The body was meant to move. There is almost always some form of exercise you can do safely. Maybe you won't be running the Boston Marathon anytime soon, but water aerobics with a yoga chaser might be the answer. Think this through if you have limitations you've been using as excuses. Write down a few forms of exercise you could actually do.

Exercise I could do: ________________________________

____

____

____

Meditation

Truth

Rising

Above

Indwelling

Negativity

Tip #1

Chocolate can Help You Lose Weight

I'm not kidding. It's all about what kind and how much. Dark chocolate contains oleoylethanolamide, better known as OEA. OEA speeds up your metabolism, increases satiety, and cools inflammation—all things that help prevent obesity. You just have to train yourself to eat a square or two, not a bar or two, of dark chocolate daily.

Two

Playing versus Exercising

When you were a child and went out to play, what did you do? Most of us were bouncing balls, jumping rope, and racing through the neighborhood playing tag. When the streetlights came on, you'd beg Mom for five more minutes, just five more minutes. As an adult, when you go out to exercise, what do you do? Many people chose the most boring thing on the planet—an exercise machine in a windowless room. They plod through their workout muttering, "Five more minutes, only five more minutes."

Nowadays we pay big money for someone to yell at us while we bounce balls, jump rope, and race around. We call it boot camp. Why do we no longer equate exercise with play? According to the American Council on Exercise, the primary reasons adults give for not exercising regularly are: boredom, lack of results, injuries, and lack of time.[1] Let's address each one and see if we can put the play back into your day.

[1] Bryant, C.X., (2007 Mar/Apr) Chief science officer. *Fitness Matters, 13,* 14.

Boredom and Lack of Results

I'm going to address these two together because I believe they are related. If the exercise you've chosen is boring, and the only reason you are doing it is to lose weight or get "vanity" muscles, you probably won't stick with it. It might be okay for a while, but honestly, unless you're 23 you're probably not going to look like a Victoria Secret model or Arnold Schwarzenegger in his heyday just from exercising. Exercise is one component of a healthy lifestyle. It can't be isolated and expected to do miracles.

What if you tackled this a different way and started to explore activities you might really like to do? A friend of mine began playing tennis, and she really looked forward to her training sessions. As she progressed in her sport, she joined a league. Because of the competition, she became interested in improving her game.

My friend did a little research. She discovered if she improved her aerobic capacity and her running skills, it would give her an edge. So, she hit the trail with a training goal in mind, and running was no longer boring. When she saw the great results running had on her game, she was inspired to go to the gym two days a week to improve her swing with strength training.

One day she put on her tennis shorts, and they fell off because she had lost so much weight. She played her way to her desired end and in the process discovered a new joy in life that will stay with her for years.

Lack of Time

When you are just starting out on your fitness adventure, you may have difficulty finding the time for exercise. A wise person once said, "If you plan nothing, that's exactly what you get." If you are not in a routine and you think you'll just exercise when you have time this week, it won't happen. This is a recipe for failure leading to guilt, despair, and self-doubt. Don't do this to yourself.

Go to your calendar every week and schedule your workouts thoughtfully taking all your week's commitments into consideration. These appointments are important. Take them just as seriously as a you would a dentist appointment. Don't argue with yourself. Don't let other people sidetrack you. Just do it.

If you aren't sure where or how to begin an activity that sounds like fun, let your motive for exercise be preparation for play. Start working on general conditioning. No exercise is fun if you are out of shape.

Injuries

People who are involved in sports occasionally get injured. There are things you can do to decrease the risk, but it does happen. I look at it this way: shin splints are better than heart disease, diabetes, high blood pressure, and obesity. The key is to play smart. Following are several hints for avoiding injuries.

1. Give your body time to adapt. You need to increase the time and intensity of your workouts incrementally. Weekend warriors are at very high risk for injury. You can't just jump back into your college swim workout after 15 years of being sedentary.

2. A good warm up before exercise and a stretch afterwords is very important. Make sure you stretch all the muscles you used.

3. Having the proper equipment is crucial, particularly the right shoes. Spend a little extra at the sports equipment store and a little less at the doctor's office.

4. Core strength training and general strength training play an important part in injury prevention as well. If your muscles get out of balance because all you do is one activity, you will be more prone to injuries.

5. Make sure you are getting enough protein in your diet. Protein is the body's muscle repair kit.

Getting Started

When people are just getting into exercise, I usually suggest starting with some kind of aerobic, or cardiovascular, activity. There are several reasons for this. If you are out of condition, any exercise ends up being a strength training exercise. Walking up a big hill may wind you, (cardiovascular exercise) but you will probably feel your legs burning by the time you reach the top as well (strength training exercise). By using your muscles functionally, as you do when you're hiking, biking, or swimming, you will prepare your body for more focused strength training in the future.

Another reason to start with aerobic exercise is it's more fun. Most people would rather go dancing, go for a brisk walk, or play racquetball than lift weights. When you exercise aerobically your body produces endorphins which are affectionately called "happy hormones" by those of us addicted to them.

Many people tell me they hate to exercise. They don't like to sweat. They feel like they're having a heart attack, asthma attack, and panic attack all rolled into one when their heart rate starts to rise. Provided you really aren't experiencing any of the above, keep at the exercise thing, and eventually your body will adapt. You'll be able to work at higher heart rates with less discomfort.

Then the endorphins will kick in. You will begin to enjoy what you're doing. Not only will you enjoy it, but you will also find you get really cranky when you can't exercise for some reason.

The situation will reverse. Instead of feeling guilty you're sitting on the couch again, you'll feel guilty because you spent too much time at the gym, in the pool, or on the trail. Be patient. For this transition to take place it will take a commitment of thirty minutes to an hour of aerobic activity at least three times a week for six weeks.

Just to tide you over until you morph into an exercise machine, here are some of the benefits:

- Reduction in blood pressure
- Increased HDL cholesterol
- Decreased total cholesterol
- Decreased body fat stores
- Increased aerobic work capacity because of the following: increased heart volume, stroke volume, cardiac output, oxygen consumption, capillary density and blood flow to active muscles, total blood volume, and lung capacity.
- Decreased anxiety and depression
- Decreased incidence of some cancers
- Increased insulin sensitivity

Not only that, but you can use a good workout to justify a piece of chocolate.

Meditate On It

Close your eyes and think back to a time when you were involved in a physical activity you enjoyed. Now think about other sports or activities you have always admired.

With these in mind, imagine your body being lithe and coordinated. See yourself flowing through the motions of these sports with ease and finesse. Think of the sounds you would hear: your breath, a ball bouncing, water splashing, or footfalls on the road. Imagine the physical sensations of sweat rolling down between your shoulder blades, the wax of a surfboard under your chest, or the light pressure of a dancing partner's hands on your back and hand. Imagine the smells of sweat, chlorine, or pine needles crunching underfoot.

Journal Work:

Write down the activity that came to mind first.

____

____

____

____

____

Write down 2 or 3 other activities you would like to do.

____

____

____

____

____

What has stopped you from participating in these activities in the past?

____

____

____

____

____

Brainstorm:

How can you fit at least one of these activities into your life once a week?

____

____

____

How can you fit in another at least once a month?

____

____

____

How about the third once a year?

____

____

____

Meditation

The Rocket Ship Rule states there is always a disproportionate amount of energy needed at the start of a new project. Once the rocket ship leaves the Earth's gravitational pull, the booster engines fall off and the ship will travel great distances with much less fuel than it took for the blast off. In other words, stick with it. It will get easier.

Tip #2

Chocolate is Good for Your Heart

Numerous studies support the assertion that the antioxidant properties of chocolate help lower LDL cholesterol, increase HDL cholesterol, lower blood sugar levels, and increase blood flow to the brain and heart. When you complete your workouts, reward yourself with a some dark chocolate.

Three

Entrepreneurial Eating Versus Defeatist Dieting

I sat down to write this chapter and, honestly, I had to get up and get something to eat. Just hearing the word "diet" makes me feel rebellious and ravenous. I was a dance minor in college so I understand something about the eternal quest for the size zero jeans. It's not only impossible for most, it's unhealthy on so many levels.

I have gone on almost every diet on the books: from cabbage soup to grapefruit, low fat to low carb, extreme calorie restriction to eat-what-you-want-but-exercise-it-off. I've taken all the latest, greatest supplements. And, I have come to the conclusion diets are disasters.

You would think because of my personal experience, and because clients actually paid me to help them lose weight, people would believe me when I tell them diets are disasters. But, often, they don't. They tell me about the diet that worked for them. "I lost 15 pounds in two weeks," they say.

"So, why are you here?" I ask.

"I gained it back. I guess I have no self-control."

Let me say right here, self-control is usually not the issue for regular dieters. Some of my most lovely, intelligent, devoted, and disciplined clients were those who'd lost the same 15 to 50 pounds over and over again. They were able to eat nothing but food looking like something invented by NASA for moon missions for months at a time.

The naturally skinny folks, on the other hand, were the ones who struggled most with self-control. They'd hit 50 and suddenly sprout love-handles. Even though they'd spent most of their lives feeling superior to heavier people, they tended to fall apart when told they had to give up a their nightly bowl of ice cream.

For the purposes of this book the definition of a Diet is: ***an artificially imposed, temporary eating pattern designed to accomplish a physical change, usually weight loss.***

When I say diet, I don't mean just cutting back a little because you're recovering from too much holiday cheer. I mean the kind of diet you could never live on. My opinion is, these type of diets are disasters and I have science on my side.

According to a multitude of sources and studies, when you go on a very restrictive diet, you go into survival mode. Face it, your body isn't the brightest bulb on the tree. It assumes the worst when you stop eating. The Mongols have invaded. There is worldwide famine. Baskin and Robins has gone out of business. Whatever it is, it must be bad.

One of the first things your body does is lower your metabolism—just what you don't want. If you're only going to feed it 800 calories a day, it will do it's best to live on that. When you come off the diet, you will regain weight rapidly. Training can work in your favor or against you, but it works.

Because there aren't enough carbohydrates coming in

while you're on a restricted diet, you begin to burn your fat reserves. That's good, right? That would be good if it stopped there, but it doesn't. You will also begin to burn muscle mass. The less muscle mass you have the lower your metabolism will be. Do you sense a trend? Your body is doing everything it can to adapt to this new situation. In some cases, your body may actually begin to burn vital organs.

Lower muscle mass and the restriction of healthy carbohydrates will decrease your ability to exercise. There are a multitude of studies that suggest exercise is instrumental in both fat loss and the ability to keep excess weight off. For those of you who think you will lose weight first then add exercise into your life, as much as 25% of the weight you lose will come from your lean muscle mass.

Here is a list of possible outcomes from restricted calorie or restricted food type—low fat, no carbohydrate, no wine or chocolate—diets:

- gallstones
- anemia
- increased risk of osteoporosis
- bloodshot eyes
- dehydration
- mineral imbalances
- vitamin deficiencies
- menstrual irregularities
- infertility
- decreased sex drive
- irritability
- sleep disorders
- depression

Health and fitness is about working with your body, not punishing it. There is a better path to a leaner, more attractive you than restrictive dieting. I like to call it *entrepreneurial eating*. According to Webster's an entrepreneur is: *one who organizes, manages and assumes the risk of an enterprise.* If we apply that definition to someone who takes control of their own weight and health, we come up with an interesting contrast to the diet mentality. Following are the some of the traits of both.

Entrepreneurial Eater:

- You are constantly evolving
- You see eating habits as unique to each individual
- You accept personal responsibility
- You are thoughtful and involved
- You take the best from many sources
- Health is your measure of success
- Your reward is nourishment and enjoyment
- You are motivated by a positive self-image
- You accept and work with reality

Defeatist Dieter

- You follow a stagnant, predetermined set of rules
- You follow a one-size-fits-all plan
- You blame or praise the diet for failure or success
- You are mindlessly obedient
- You rely on one source
- The scale is your measure of success
- Your punishment is deprivation and guilt
- You are motivated by a poor body image
- You often foster unrealistic expectations

If you find yourself falling into the *defeatist dieter* mentality, you are not alone. This kind of thinking is the environment in which eating disorders are born. Unfortunately, it is all too common in our culture. Recognizing negative thinking patterns is the first step to rising above them and learning to mind your own body.

Nutritional Basics:

If you are going to take charge in the eating department, you're going to have to learn some basic nutritional information. There are three categories of macro-nutrients: protein, carbohydrates and fats. Most foods contain some of each but tend to be grouped into categories based on what they contain the most of.

- **Protein foods**: Meat, poultry, fish, eggs, dairy, legumes, and nuts
- **Carbohydrate foods:** Grains, vegetables, and fruit
- **High Fat foods:** Oils, nut butters, and products from animal fat such as butter and lard.

Many diets revolve around arranging these macro-nutrients in certain percentages or trying to all but eliminate one or the other. Your body needs them all, but how much of each is unique to each individual's situation.

If you're an athlete in training, you will need extra protein to repair and build your muscles. If you have insulin resistance, which is becoming increasingly prevalent, you will have to seriously restrict your carbohydrates and carefully chose the type of carbohydrates you eat. Certain body types do better with certain mixes of macro-nutrients and, of course, we have to take into account your personal likes and dislikes. This will be a process of discovery as you apply what you learn.

There are, however, general rules that hold true for everybody. The easiest formula is to try to eat food as close to the way God created it as possible. If you have a choice between brown or white rice, chose brown. If you have a choice between grass fed beef or corn fed, hormone pumped beef, choose grass fed. Fish should be wild not farmed. Vegetables and fruit should be organic whenever possible.

If a food has a whole lot of ingredients on the label you can't pronounce or draw a picture of, don't eat it. Eat as many fresh, non-starchy vegetables as possible in a day. If all this sounds hard, remember, we are training. No one is expecting perfection overnight—except maybe you.

You may find yourself having sugar or carbohydrate cravings as you begin to change your eating habits. High fructose corn syrup and other high sugar foods have an addictive effect on our bodies. We have to either go cold turkey or wean ourselves from these foods. Following are some ideas to help the process.

Tips for overcoming sugar cravings:

- Eat 5 to 6 small meals, or 3 meals and 2 to 3 snacks a day
- Avoid simple carbohydrates
- Do cardiovascular exercise regularly
- Eat lots of non-starchy vegetables
- Get plenty of rest

Some herbs, spices, and supplements that may help are:

- Cinnamon
- Turmeric
- American Ginseng
- Flaxseed
- Fenugreek
- Chromium Picolinate

Another problem we run into when we focus on a restrictive diet is we tend to be hungry all the time. If you are not getting enough micro-nutrients, your diet might fill your stomach, but it won't give you the nutrition you need. As soon as your stomach is empty (usually about 15 minutes), you begin to feel hungry again.

If you hardly ever eat fruits and vegetables, when your body is in dire need of vitamins A and C it doesn't know where to go for those nutrients. You will just crave more food. The better your diet is, the more educated your body becomes. When it's in need of vitamin C, it will crave an orange or broccoli. So, wrapping this up, remember your new mindset is: *high quality nourishment is good. Depriving myself is bad.*

Meditation

"A diet is a plan, generally hopeless, for reducing your weight, which tests your will power but does little for your waistline."
- Herbert B. Prochnow

TIP #3

How to Choose Chocolate

Not all chocolate is created equal. Sorry, but a Snickers isn't going to do much for your waistline or your health. You've got to read the label. Following are a few things to look for:

- a minimal amount of added sugar (cane sugar is best)
- no cocoa butter equivalents (CBE)
- 70% cocoa or more
- organic or free trade sources
- no Dutching*

Cocoa nibs are a great way to get the most out of your chocolate. (Check the resources pages at the back of the book for more chocolate education and places to purchase.)

*Dutching is a method of processing cocoa invented in 1828 by a Dutch chocolatier using pressure and alkaline salts. Although this was very entrepreneurial of Van Houten, the process removes much of chocolate's healthy properties.

THIS IS THE END OF THE FIRST MESOCYCLE.

Spend a week settling into your new habits and have some wine and chocolate.

Why I Love Wine

"Wine is the thinking person's health drink." - Dr. Phillip Norrie

For those of us who love wine, it is much more than a beverage. It's a lifestyle. What is more soothing to the soul than wandering around a pastoral vineyard embracing the sights, sounds, smells, and tastes? The wine experience not only incorporates all the senses, it elicits feelings of joy and generosity. The Bible says, "God made wine to make the heart glad." And, that it does. Anything that involves so much pleasure must be good for you, right? I would argue wine is good for you on many levels, and the scientific community backs me up.

For thousands of years the health benefits of wine were common knowledge. Medical journals regularly listed its pharmaceutical attributes. The alcohol and acids in wine killed many of the bacteria and parasites in drinking water. A mix of the two was considered a safer drink than pure water. The sedative and euphoric effects of wine were also utilized to help those with anxiety or depression. It was applied topically as an antiseptic.

During Prohibition wine became a forbidden drink, and its usefulness was erased from the medical journals. Prohibitionists were fighting the cultural effects of alcoholism. Of course overindulgence in anything is not good for anyone. Too much food makes you obese; too much exercise leads to injury; even too much water can lead to death. This obvious perspective was overlooked, and wine was lumped in with rot-gut liquor and moonshine.

Recently, health experts have been re-exploring the benefits of wine. Their findings are almost as euphoria producing as the wine itself. A glass or two of vino a day can prolong life, decrease the likelihood of dementia or Alzheimer's, lower cholesterol and the risk of stroke and coronary disease, reduce the risks of certain cancers, and even help you fight the common cold.

Other studies have shown wine drinking women tend to have higher bone density than non-drinking women. Wine boosts estrogen levels which helps to maintain healthy bones after menopause. I'm headed to the kitchen. I'm sure I have a bottle of something open.

Mesocycle Two

Gaining Thin Thoughts

Your goal for the next three weeks is to begin to take charge of your wayward inner child. You're now armed with the information you need to make positive changes, both physically and mentally. Here are your action steps.

Meditation Exercise - Get Educated

Go back to your *Meditate On It* page in chapter two. What sports or activities did you write down? Research groups in your area that promote those activities. Go to a Meet Up, coaching meeting, order a book or a magazine, sign up for a race, or get a guest pass to a gym. Do you know anyone who's doing what you're interested in? Call them this week and see what kind of advice they can give you to help you get started.

Getting involved with others who are doing what you're interested in is key to your success. Remember the cheerleaders we talked about in chapter one? You're taking the first steps to create your support team.

Journal Work:

Write down who you're going to contact and when.

Moderation Exercise - Kitchen Cleanse:

You've been keeping a food diary for a month. You know what you *have* been eating, but what *should* you be eating? Remember, I said real food is not bad. Chemicals and overly processed foods are not real food. You have to begin to eliminate them from your diet and replace them with what they originally replaced. You're going back to your food roots. A kitchen cleanse is a practical way to start the process.

Journal Work:

Go through your pantry, fridge, and cupboards. Make a list of any foods you find containing the following:

- Enriched wheat flour
- High Fructose Corn Syrup
- Trans fats
- Hydrogenated or partially hydrogenated oils
- Artificial sweeteners (Stevia's okay)
- Food coloring
- Artificial flavors
- Monosodium Glutamate
- Sodium Nitrate/Sodium Nitrite
- BHA and BHT
- Sulfur Dioxide
- Potassium Bromate

Take this list to your local, healthier food market. Whole Foods, Mother's, Sprouts, Trader Joes, and farmer's markets are all good options. Look for replacement products that don't contain anything from the "banned" list. Box up all your "banned foods" and send them to the local food bank. From now on purchase from your new and improved food list.

If portion control is still a problem for you, continue with your food diary. If you are staying within your allotted calories fairly easily on most days, you can discontinue food tracking. Food tracking is a great tool to use when you come off a holiday period, or anytime your eating habits get out of hand.

Acceleration Exercise - Schedule It

Remember, if you plan for nothing, that's exactly what you'll get. Think through your week. What commitments do you have? Where can you fit in some play time to get your body moving? Even if you're not ready to start your new sport or activity, plan some time to prep your body for what's coming.

Journal Work:

For the next three weeks schedule your exercise appointments. You can do this below or on a calendar, whatever works best for you. If you haven't been exercising at all, or if you haven't been doing any cardiovascular exercise, make sure you plan at least 4 to 5 sessions of cardiovascular exercise a week. Include what you're going to do, what time you are going to do it, and how long it will take.

Sunday	Monday	Tuesday	Wednesday	Thursday	Friday	Saturday

Four

Slowing Down to Get Ahead

I am a cardio queen. Take me running, swimming, dancing, and even strength training, as long as I can do it to a beat and get my heart rate up. Slowing down is hard for me. However, I have watched clients throw themselves into a flurry of activity attempting to change their bodies overnight only to wind up frustrated and injured. I'm the last one to tell you to spend a lot of time on the couch, but sometimes the best way to get ahead is to slow down.

This week I'd like you to take some time to set long-term goals and ponder the baby steps it will take to reach them. Think ahead to where you want to be ten years from now, five years in the future, and next year this time. Take into consideration your time constraints, physical constraints, financial constraints, family constraints, and even character constraints. Assume roadblocks will come up. Give yourself plenty of time to accomplish what you want to accomplish.

I realize this is difficult when you are all pumped up about starting a new lifestyle. You believe those who do it fastest are the rising stars. Your impatience to get in shape will urge you to skip all kinds of steps, to find the shortcuts you think only the really bright and edgy know about.

Several years ago a man wanted to hire me as a personal trainer—for ten minutes a week. He brought me a book claiming that's all you needed to be in the best shape of your life. The model on the cover looked like Mr. America. This ten minute workout was supposed to increase your muscle tone, give you a great cardiovascular system, and help you lose all your unwanted fat. It sounded too good to be true. It was. Fitness fads and gimmicks come and go. Remember, you're in it for the long haul.

Goal Setting:

There are lots of things to think about when goal setting. I've heard and observed people tend to be more successful when they think like an overachiever in the long term but like an underachiever in the short term. Remember, ***training employs small steps to reach audacious goals.***

So dream big, but give yourself plenty of time to get there. This is especially true when it comes to fitness. You should leave most workouts feeling tired, but energized and excited about the next one. The weekend warrior syndrome is very common, but it often leads to injuries and failure.

Is your primary goal weight loss? If you have a very high BMI (body mass index), you may definitely need to lose weight, but setting a specific number of pounds as your goal can backfire on you. How much weight your body chooses to lose in response to a change in diet and exercise isn't something you have control over.

Some people will lose weight like crazy at first, then plateau. Others can't seem to lose a pound for months then, finally, begin to lose. Others only lose a negligible amount of weight but drop four sizes and look and feel terrific.

Weight loss doesn't always equate to better fitness. Muscle tissue is heavier than fat. Your bones increase in density as you strength train. These things can make you heavier.

The other problem I have with making weight loss your goal is a psychological one. Marcia Weider says in her book *Making Your Dreams Come True,*[1] "There's a different kind of energy involved when moving toward what you want than there is when moving away from what you don't want."

One is a positive energy using momentum to move you forward. The other is negative energy that only drives you so far. As soon as you begin to feel comfortable again, you tend to slip back into the old ways that got you into trouble in the first place. You didn't create a new you, a new adventure, a new perspective. You were just troubleshooting the old one.

My Dad once gave me a great analogy that applies to much in life. Remember those multi-step math problems we had to do in high school? What if you got one or two steps wrong right in the middle of long division? You couldn't just keep going and say to yourself, "I'll do it right from here on in." It wouldn't work. You'd end up with the wrong answer. You'd have to ditch the work and start over to get it right. The moral of the story: Sometimes you can't just fix the problem. You have to create something new in your life.

I encourage clients to set goals they can dream about. Becoming or doing something is exciting. Becoming a runner, a triathlete, a health-food chef, or a fashionista in a size six is heady stuff. You can subscribe to magazines, find new friends with like interests and talk about your hobby until old friends get irritated. The more consumed and fascinated you become, the less you will think about your waistline,

---

[1]Weider, Marcia. *Making Your Dreams Come True.* New York: Harmony Books, 1999

and the quicker it will shrink.

Have you ever noticed how disciplined people get when they want to look good for an upcoming event? That's because they are visualizing themselves entering the room and impressing everyone in attendance with how attractive they are. The problem is once the event is over, so is the discipline. Visualizing yourself as a healthy and fit individual defined by a new, long-term interest is a much better solution.

Meditate On It

A common goal setting technique is to utilize the acronym SMART. The letters stand for specific, measurable, attainable, relevant and time-bound. This is a great way to analyze and create a reasonable plan for your fitness program. Let's go through them one by one.

Specific – Goals must have definition in order for us to know how to reach them. If my goal is to climb a mountain, I must first decide if I'm talking about a small, one day climb or Kilimanjaro. My training and preparation would look entirely different for each. "I want to get in shape," or "I want to lose weight," are not specific goals. They are impossible to plan for.

Measurable – The goal must have parameters. If you're planning to climb a local mountain, you'd better know the route's distance and incline. If you don't know where the top is, how can you say, "I've arrived"?

Attainable – You must be realistic. On her first personal training appointment, A 50-year-old, overweight woman announced she wanted me to make her look like Jennifer Lopez. This wasn't going to happen. Whatever goals you set must include you at the end of them.

Relevant – Your goals must be relevant to your life. If you are already so busy you can barely find time to brush your teeth, running a marathon may not be a good choice. A series of 10K races would be much better since the training is less time consuming.

Time-bound – Goals must have calendar dates attached to them. If they don't, we have a terrible way of procrastinating until we lose our enthusiasm. When that happens, our goals are never reached. Make sure your time table takes all the small steps into consideration.

Journal Work:

What do you want to accomplish through this training? Write out your SMART goal. Specifically, what is it? What are its measurable qualities? How will you know when you've reached it? Think hard, is it relevant to your life? Do you need to tweak it a little to make it more realistic? What are the potential road blocks you may face and how can you work around them? Finally, put some dates on it. When is your deadline? What are the dates you expect to have the smaller steps accomplished by? Add these dates to your calendar, or workout schedule.

Specific - ____________________

Measurable - ____________________

Attainable - ____________________

Relevant - ____________________

Time-bound - ____________________

Sunday	Monday	Tuesday	Wednesday	Thursday	Friday	Saturday

Tip #4

Chocolate Will Make You Happy

Chocolate has natural mood enhancing compounds. It contains *Phenethylamine* (PEA), which boosts opioid levels in your brain. *Opioids,* like their chemical cousins, opiates, work as pain relievers and confidence and pleasure enhancers. Chocolate also contains *Tryptophan,* which promotes serotonin production. Serotonin helps you stay relaxed and calm.

FIVE
Bouncing or Splatting?

If I throw down a Super Ball, it bounces right back up at me. If I throw down a Hacky Sack, it splats. This demonstrates the difference between a strong, solid core and a soft, mushy center.

Core is a popular word in the fitness industry. You've probably seen all kinds of cute and clever class names like *Core and More, Core Training,* and the *Core Issue.* Maybe you've been wondering what they're all about. To demystify, the core is your torso. It includes everything but your head and limbs. It contains the spinal column, which represents your mid-line and protects the nerves innervating every area of your body. It contains your internal organs, which are protected by your rib cage, pelvic girdle, and the surrounding musculature.

As you can see, it is a very important part of your body and deserves more attention than a few crunches a week. Everything you do is done with more energy, less effort, and greater strength if you have a Super Ball core. Since all movement involves the center of your body to one degree or another, a core that is out of balance with the rest of your muscles is an injury waiting to happen.

Paul Bragg, who was Jack LaLanne's mentor, would invite people to jump on his abs in his exercise classes. This, by the way, when he was in his eighties. He did it to prove the point—a strong core protects the internal organs. I'm not recommending that. However, if we look back at some of the grandfathers of the fitness industry—Paul Bragg, Jack LaLanne and Joseph Pilates—their strength and agility at advanced ages is a testimonial to the importance of developing this area of the body.

How many people over the age of 45 do you know with a back problem? Probably a lot. Back problems are epidemic in our country and are exacerbated by weak abdominal muscles, poor posture, and carrying too much weight. Many back problems can be completely reversed by strengthening core muscles and taking off a few pounds.

A strong core will transfer muscular forces from the limbs throughout the body. This allows you to run faster, jump higher, and leap tall buildings in a single bound. Well, not the tall building part, but it will definitely help you lift heavier weight more safely. It will improve your balance, coordination, and ability to swing or throw with force. A strong core also acts as a shock absorber, helping to protect the feet, ankles, and knees from injury.

Flexibility:

Another thing these supermen of the fitness industry understood was the importance of flexibility training. When we participate in an activity, the muscles we use will be strengthened. When muscles are strengthened, they get shorter unless we counteract that by stretching them. Shortened muscles can cause postural problems resulting in injury or chronic pain. Training opposing muscles is part of the fix. We'll talk more about that in the chapter on strength training. Another component is flexibility training, or stretching.

Tight hamstrings are a common problem. They're caused

by walking, running, climbing stairs, and many day to day activities. Over time, short, tight hamstrings can lead to postural problems. Stretching the legs correctly will lengthen the hamstrings and that, plus strengthening the core muscles, can alleviate back pain.

I had been an avid runner for a number of years. I took a break while I was pregnant. After the birth of my daughter, I tried to return to my normal workout schedule. But, after a few weeks of training, my back would go out.

The strain my back muscles and the stretching my abdominal muscles endured during pregnancy made them unable to withstand the tightening of my hamstrings. I would end up on the couch in pain with ice packs on my back.

Obviously, with two small children this couldn't go on. I had to give up running. About ten years later, I began teaching Pilates mat classes. I could feel it changing my body.

One day, a student asked me to go for a run with her. I told her my sad, back story and her response was, "Have you tried running since you've been doing Pilates?" I hadn't. Silly me. I went for a run with her and ten years and many half marathons later, I'm still running.

In your next mesocycle, you'll be challenged to include some core training into your life. Begin thinking about ways you could do it. Classes, videos, or working on your own are all options.

Meditation

"A fat stomach sticks out too far. It prevents you from looking down and seeing what is going on around you."
- Norman Reilly Raine

Tip #5

Chocolate is a Stimulant

Chocolate wakes you up and can cure your cough, but it can also kill Fido. It contains several mild stimulants: caffeine, phenylethylamine, anandamide and theobromine.

Most cultures love their stimulants. The Brits and the Chinese have tea. Swedes and Americans can't live without coffee. The Mayans were addicted to cocoa. Chocolate was so important to the ancients, the beans were used for currency, and the drink was a part of their religious ceremonies.

Theobromine, one of those stimulants, can be fatal to your dog. Animals don't have the enzymes needed to metabolize it. Even a small amount of chocolate can make your pooch very sick. However, theobromine is very effective for treating a persistent cough in people. Try sucking on a square of dark chocolate instead of a cough drop next flu season

Six
Educating Your Palate

If I took you shopping and we went to a store that had clothing the quality of Walmart's but was priced like Nordstrom's, you'd look at me like I was crazy. This analogy applies well to food. Most people who are overweight are eating Walmart food at Nordstrom prices.

Let's imagine you have a certain number of calories to spend every day. For those calories you ought to have so much protein, so much complex carbohydrate, so many micro-nutrients, so much fiber, and so on. Why would you spend those calories on foods that had a very high price tag but were very low-quality? "Because I like them," you say. But, what if I could take you to a store that had great quality clothes at Walmart prices? Would you consider shopping there?

Many of the foods you enjoy can be "purchased" much more cheaply. A Big Mac at McDonald's has 29 grams of unhealthy animal fat, fillers and preservatives, a white bread bun, trans fat laden salad dressing and cheese, and 25 grams of protein. It will cost you 540 calories. A burger made at home with 95% lean ground, grass fed, hormone-free beef has only 5 grams of fat and still has 25 grams of protein for 125 calorie cost. If you add a whole grain bun, you up your price to 225 calories, but you're adding complex carbohydrates, a little more protein, and fiber. You can also add a salad dressing containing healthy fats for less calories.

I understand making dietary changes can be very upsetting. We like our ruts. But, remember the training principles from chapter one. You can do this a little at a time. You can retrain your eating habits.

Training means making small changes with consistency and allowing yourself to physically and mentally adapt before another change is introduced.

Have you ever had a dog? Generally, dogs eat the same food day after day, year after year. Do you know what happens when you change their dog food to another brand? It's not pretty.

My neighbor gave me a bag of dog food her dog wouldn't eat. That should have waved a few red flags, but I gave it to my dog without thinking. The poor thing got horrible diarrhea. The lethal smelling flatulence is something I will never forget.

When I decided to put her on senior formula food years later, I had learned my lesson. This time I did it gradually. I mixed her current food with increasingly larger amounts of the new food, until she was eating senior formula exclusively. Everyone was much happier. All that to say, I don't want you to go out and radically change your diet this week. I am hoping, however, over the course of this program you will have made radical dietary changes.

Part of the problem is, often, we're not educated. We don't realize what we're eating. There is a direct correlation in our country between the size of our wallets and the size of our waistbands. I believe this is an educational issue. Generally speaking, people in higher income brackets have been taught more and therefore make better choices.

Back to the clothing analogy, I love the show *What Not to Wear*. Stacy and Clinton take people who are wearing very low quality clothing and teach them to appreciate beautiful clothes that fit and work well for them. The candidates usually begin the program defending the merits of their old wardrobe. By the end, they realize how much better the new clothes really are.

Don't defend a poor diet. Save yourself the embarrassment of having to eat your words. Your body will respond to high-quality food over time just as the candidates on *What Not to Wear* finally respond to their new look.

As I've stated before, taste is learned. You usually like what you were raised on. Likes and dislikes can change as your appreciation grows. Training principal #2 applies well here.

Training will actually alter the physical makeup of your body, change your emotional state, and give you knowledge you can't unlearn.

Food preferences are learned. Some cultures eat bugs, and they like them. Some eat cabbage that has been buried in the ground for two months, and they like it. Some people don't like chocolate. Weird, I know.

You can learn to like vegetables. Over time your tastes will adapt to a new diet. You will lose preferences for certain foods and gain preferences for others. I had a client who changed her eating habits pretty drastically during the time we worked together. When Thanksgiving came, she went to a relative's for dinner and had the usual fat laden fare. She felt like she was suffering from a severe hangover for several days after. It wasn't pleasant. Even if certain foods still taste good to you, if they make you feel sick they will begin to lose their allure. Trust the process.

Sometimes my clients complain this all takes too much time. Eating well, ultimately, does not take any more time than eating poorly; it just takes the application of training principal #3. Change is time-consuming, but once you make the new grocery list, create the new recipes, find the right stores and restaurants, you'll be in your new groove. The *Meditate On It* page for this chapter will provide some tools to help you through the process painlessly.

Training disciplines your body, working with it to bring out your natural strengths and abilities; it is not about punishment.

The goal is to make changes in your eating habits in a slow, progressive, and consistent manner. The changes should become a part of your life pattern. Wouldn't it be wonderful if eating healthy wasn't something you had to think about all the time? A diet make-over is a creative process. It should highlight your particular talents in the kitchen and your likes and dislikes. You will learn to strengthen your body with the foods it needs.

Don't fret about it. You have the rest of your life to get it right. Diets punish and deprive. Changing your habits is a loving thing to do for yourself and for your family.

Meditate On It

Many of us have unhealthy, emotional attachments to foods we should only be eating small amounts of. I know you're thinking, "What about you with your wine and chocolate, Greta?" You are right—at least you were. I've had to do some soul searching and put my treats into their appropriate place in my life. There was a time when the thought of going without a couple of brownies at lunch would get me all choked up.

A treat is something you celebrate with, not something you medicate with. A treat is something you thoughtfully choose, not something you can't resist. Any foods containing things from the banned ingredient list, "white" stuff (white flour, white sugar, white rice, white potatoes), alcohol, or high levels of animal fat should be considered treats.

Journal Work:

Write down any foods you feel may have an unhealthy hold on you.

____

____

____

When are you most susceptible to indulging in these foods?

____

____

____

If you tell yourself you can never have this food again, or try to drastically reduce how often you eat it, the craving may grow worse. Here's a psychological trick to try if you're struggling with self-control.

Allow yourself to eat this food whenever you want, but change the place or circumstances. If you have to have a Snicker's Bar every day, you can have it. But, you have to eat it in the bathtub or shower stall. If you have to have a bowl of ice cream every night before bed, make yourself eat it standing in the front yard while wearing your bathrobe. If, instead, you chose a square of dark chocolate or an apple, you can eat those in the same place or circumstances you would have eaten the Snicker's bar or ice cream.

Write out your new rules:

Foods to limit:

Where/how if I want to indulge?

When can I treat myself?

How much can I have?

Meditation

"No diet will remove all the fat from your body because the brain is entirely fat. Without a brain, you might look good, but all you could do is run for public office." - George Bernard Shaw

Tip #6

Chocolate Will Make You Smarter

According to a study done at Northumbria University, U.K., the flavanols in chocolate increase mental acuity by promoting blood flow to the brain. Epicatechin, a chocolate compound, was shown to improve the memories of mice and protect their brains from the effects of strokes in experiments done at the Salk Institute of California. Try some dark chocolate next time you need to study for a test.

You have now finished Mesocycle Two.

Take a week to ponder your navel, practice what you've learned, and own your new habits. Don't forget to have some wine and chocolate.

Wine Makes You Thinner - Really

"I cook with wine, sometimes I even add it to the food."
- W. C. Fields

Did you know the average wine drinker, when compared with the rest of the population, has a smaller waistline, less belly fat, and lower body mass? Not only that, but they tend to be better educated, have a higher IQ, eat more fruits and vegetables, and exercise more.

Now, I know what you're thinking—along with how much you like me right now. You're thinking, wine drinkers' lifestyles are better, ergo they are thinner. Maybe, but which comes first the grape or the seed?

I certainly agree, living la vida vino includes a number of health producing benefits. Having a more educated palate would make you more discerning about food choices. Enjoying the bounty of nature and living close to the land are part of loving wine. These are all things that improve health.

You can, however, be fit and fat. I have worked with many foodies, triathletes, swimmers, and vegetarian Yogis who were just that. So, it seems there may be a quality in wine itself that helps to keep us from middle-aged spread.

A thirteen year study was done by Brigham and Women's Hospital in Boston[1]. In this study they tracked the drinking habits of women. It turns out, women who drink moderately have a 30 percent lower chance of weight gain. When wine was specifically targeted, the results were even more dramatic.

A Swiss study showed digestion was improved and slowed when a heavy meal was paired with white wine versus black tea. The same study showed when people drank alcohol with a meal, they tended to eat less.

What a joyful day it was when I discovered not all calories are created equal. A team at Boston University found alcohol calories are metabolized differently than the calories from food.[2] They are quickly used and aren't stored in fat. In fact, your metabolism may actually be elevated for as long as 90 minutes after you drink a glass of wine.

If that isn't good enough news, resveritrol, the wonder ingredient found in red wine, is actually believed to destroy fat cells. Do I hear an amen? This property is being further researched because resveritrol also appears to protect the body from metabolic syndrome and diabetes, both of which are associated with obesity. The more I study the benefits of drinking wine, and the more I drink it, the happier I get.

---

[1]Wang L, Lee I, Manson JE, Buring JE, Sesso HD. *Alcohol Consumption, Weight Gain, and Risk of Becoming Overweight in Middle-aged and Older Women. Arch Intern Med.* 2010;170(5):453-461. doi:10.1001/archinternmed.2009.527.

[2]Clerc O, Nanchen D, Cornuz J, Marques-Vidal P, Gmel G, Daeppen J-B, Paccaud F, Mooser V, Waeber G, Vollenweider P, Rodondi N. *Alcohol drinking, the metabolic syndrome and diabetes in a population with high mean alcohol consumption. Diabet Med,* 2010;27

Mesocycle Three

Living Strong

Your goal for the next month is to grow stronger mentally, emotionally, and physically. In order to gain strength we have to push against the obstacles in our way.

To gain muscle mass, we have to lift or move heavy objects. To gain self-control, we have to assert ourselves in the areas we have been weakest. To gain confidence, we have to do the things that have intimidated us. This may not be the most comfortable three weeks, but it's necessary if you want to reach your goals. If you've stuck with me this far, I know you can do it.

Meditation Exercise - Performance Review

How are you doing on your goals? Have you gotten involved in a sport or physical activity? Take a little time to review your journal work and assess your progress. Sometimes as we move toward a goal, we realize we need to readjust our timetable or our expectations. The key to not feeling like a failure is to stay flexible, but not so flexible you don't accomplish anything at all.

Journal Work:

Write out any successes you've had, or mistakes you've made, in achieving your fitness goals thus far. What have you learned from them? Do you need to readjust your plans?

____

____

____

____

____

____

____

____

____

____

____

____

____

____

____

____

____

____

Moderation Exercise - Menu Planning

You've kept a food diary for at least a month. Look back at it. What are your eating patterns? A common pattern fostering weight gain is eating very little in the early part of the day when resolve is strong, then eating a lot, especially high carbohydrate foods, later in the day when fatigue has lowered your resistance to temptation.

There is no scientific evidence eating at night makes you fat. There are studies, however, showing people who eat breakfast and maintain their blood sugar levels during the day are less likely to be overweight.

Generally speaking, the best eating pattern is to eat when you are hungry, but not so hungry you lose self-control. I usually recommend eating three small meals and two to three snacks throughout the day. But if you find you're eating when you're not hungry, feel free to make adjustments. If you don't need them, snacks just add unwanted calories.

Based on what you've learned about yourself, plan your eating habits for the next month. Each meal or snack you chose to eat should contain complex carbohydrates, protein, and fat. A good snack would be an apple and a handful of raw almonds, a plain Greek yogurt with some berries and a little agave nectar or stevia, or veggie sticks and humus. I'm a big proponent of protein smoothies too, especially for those of you who have a hard time eating breakfast.

As you plan your eating patterns, take your workout schedule into consideration. You want to make sure you're having some protein within an hour of an intense workout. Also, remember one of your goals is to eat as many fresh, non-starchy vegetables as you can.

Journal Work:

Breakfast ideas

____

____

____

____

Snack #1 ideas

____

____

____

____

Lunch ideas

____

____

____

____

Snack #2 ideas

____

____

____

____

Dinner ideas

____

____

____

____

Snack #3 ideas

____

____

____

____

Most of us eat the same foods for breakfast and lunch on most days of the week, so that part should be easy. Don't feel you have to write out each meal in detail, or stick to it perfectly, but at least write down enough information to help you plan ahead. Use this exercise as a guide to help you plan your grocery list. If you're busy, be sure you have healthy, easy to grab foods on hand. If you don't you'll resort to the office snack machine or the local drive-through when you're hungry.

Acceleration Exercise - Explore the Core

Continue scheduling your workouts, but now add in a core strength component at least twice a week. This could be as simple as doing some abdominal exercises after your usual workout, or as focused as going to a Pilates class twice a week.

Sunday	Monday	Tuesday	Wednesday	Thursday	Friday	Saturday

Seven

Going Down For The Count

I know it seems funny to start out a mesocycle entitled *Living Strong* with a chapter on rest, but rest and effort are the yin and yang of strength training. Did you know your body doesn't actually gain strength while you are working out, but in the rest period *after* the workout?

While you are lifting weights, your body is actually breaking down muscle tissue. That muscle is healed and made stronger during recovery. Rest is a very deceiving thing. It seems as if you should feel guilty when you are doing it, as if nothing is happening. Nothing could be farther from the truth. Rest is a time of transformation.

There are two kinds of rest, total and active. If you find yourself completely depleted, on the edge of injury, actually injured, or mind numbingly burnt out, it is time for a total rest. Take a week off. Sleep, eat, and be merry. Go to the beach. There are times I have to refuse to think about my personal goals if I don't want to blow a fuse. I've learned to cut myself some slack and listen to my inner cry for a break. The unfortunate thing is many don't. They push through, only to end up fizzling out, feeling like a failure, and throwing their goals out the window.

I once had a client who was working very hard at making a lifestyle change. She had about 150 pounds to lose, and she started out with a bang. She met with me five days a week, gave up fast food, began counting calories, and challenged her husband's resistance to her new lifestyle. It was intense.

After two months, the whole thing began to unravel. First, she began missing one or two appointments in a week. Then she slipped back into her old fast food, drive-through routine. All of a sudden, she didn't have time to shop and cook. I recognized the signs of burnout.

She needed a break, but she was afraid. She feared she wouldn't come back. She feared this would be one more failed attempt at getting her life in shape. So, she kept pushing on. You know the end of the story. Her fear became self-fulfilling prophecy. She came and went occasionally for about one more month, and I never saw her again.

Do not be afraid of taking a break. I can't say it any more forcefully. You will sabotage your success if you let fear be your driving motivation. That kind of fear is not productive. You can be in charge of your breaks. You can decide where, when, and how long. Don't let burn out spin you out of control.

Weight lifting is a great illustration for the need to give yourself permission to rest. If we lift every day, we are constantly breaking down our muscles and never giving them a chance to repair. We will get injured, and there is no coming back from some injuries. That is why every three weeks there is a break built into this program. I'm leaving it up to you whether you need total or active rest, but I want you to rest.

Building periods of active rest into your schedule can reduce the amount of total rest time you need. There are many different ways to do this. You can change your exercise routine completely. If you've been jogging four days a week and going to Pilates two days, you could try Zumba, walking, boot camp, swimming, tennis, or whatever strikes you as fun.

Not only is this good for your psyche, but change prevents plateaus. When you do the same thing continuously, you stop making gains. Over the years, I've seen what I call *checking the box syndrome*. This is done by people who come into the gym day after day, month after month, year after year and do the same exact exercise routine. They get to check the box on their to-do list.

God bless them for being consistent. If these people are happy with their level of fitness, they are staying injury-free, and they can stand the boredom, great. However, this is not for those who want to see physical improvements. Mix it up. Another bonus is you might find something new you love to do.

Cross training, workouts or training schedules that include a variety of exercises, can also help to prevent injuries. Using our bodies in different ways works different muscle groups, rather than taxing the same muscles and joints in the same ways over and over. Whether we're talking about exercise, food intake, or mental stimulation, variety is the spice of life.

Dietary Rest

You can apply the idea of scheduled rests to your eating habits as well. Many health coaches are proponents of total rest, or periods of fasting, to cleanse the system, renew self-control, and grow in spirit. There are entire books on the subject of fasting, so I won't go into that here. I suggest doing some research before embarking on a fasting program.

An active dietary rest, or choosing a detoxifying diet for a week or two, can accomplish many of the same things as a total fast but is much easier on your lifestyle. It's hard to maintain a normal schedule when doing a total fast. (Some of the websites on my resources list at the end of the book offer detoxifying programs.)

Another way to take an active rest in regard to eating habits is to take a break from recording calories and just enjoy food for a week. You may be surprised at how your tastes have changed. Often people find when they tell themselves they can eat whatever they want, they're still choosing salad, but maybe adding a little blue cheese.

Some weight loss experts believe eating more calories now and again is a good thing. The body tends to adapt, as we've been learning. If you keep your calorie intake too low for too long, you will adapt to that new lowered intake. You'll stop losing weight unless you restrict yourself even more.

If you want this change you are working so hard to accomplish to be permanent, you are going to have to find the natural rhythms of your life and plug into them. If my goal was to swim one length in my pool, I might be able to do it on one breath. (I have a really small pool.) But as soon as I increased my goal to five or ten laps, I'd be a goner. If I want to go the distance, I have to learn a breathing rhythm: two strokes, breath, two strokes, breath. Now I can swim indefinitely.

Patterns of life are just as important. Our bodies have natural rhythms. We experience hormonal rhythms, hunger rhythms, strength and exhaustion rhythms, sleep rhythms, and on and on. The Bible says there is a time for everything, including rest. Rest is a natural part of the rhythm of life. If you try to fight it, your body will derail your plans for the sake of self-preservation. Remember, training works with your body to transform it. It isn't about punishment.

Meditate On It

Times of rest are good for reviewing and renewing. Close your eyes and relax. Focus on your breath. Take time to ponder the following questions. When you open your eyes, you can record your answers.

Journal work:

What is the most significant thing you've learned in the past two months?

____

____

____

____

In what ways have you adapted mentally and emotionally so far?

____

____

____

____

In what ways have you adapted physically so far?

____

____

____

____

In what ways have you adapted in your eating habits?

____

____

____

____

What was the most difficult change for you to make? Or, what are you the most proud of yourself for accomplishing?

____

____

____

What would you like to accomplish in the next year?

____

____

____

What fears and doubts do you have about your ability to accomplish your desires?

____

____

____

What truth can you tell yourself that will calm your fears and dispel your doubts?

____

____

____

Meditation

"Sorrow can be alleviated by good sleep, a bath and a glass of wine." - Thomas Aquinas

Tip #7

Chocolate, a Natural Sun Screen

The flavonoids in dark chocolate will help protect your skin from the U.V. rays of the sun. The protection comes from the cumulative effects of eating chocolate daily for an extended period of time. Don't expect one square to prevent a sunburn. If you go to the beach for some down time this week, you still need your sun block. But, it's nice to know you have a chocolate back-up.

EIGHT
Being Leaner And Meaner

Generally speaking, people troubled by their weight don't want to weight train. They are afraid of "bulking up" and feel it is a waste of their exercise time, because it doesn't give them the high calorie cost of a cardiovascular workout.

Women especially worry about bulking up. They're concerned they'll end up looking like Xena the Warrior Princess instead of Sleeping Beauty. Never fear. Women do not have the hormones men have, so unless they take steroids, there is only so much muscle hypertrophy that will take place. Some women will build more muscle mass than others due to their body type. However, unless a woman gets into serious bodybuilding and spends hours in the gym, she won't bulk up.

Strength training is as—or more—important than cardiovascular training for weight management. Most people begin losing muscle at about age 25. Muscle tissue is more metabolic than fat. Therefore as you lose it, your metabolism drops. A raised metabolism will burn more calories per hour regardless of what you are doing. So you will burn more calories while you're sleeping, cooking, shopping, going to work, or exercising. Also, weight training helps to prevent osteoporosis and makes you look great.

People tell me they've tried strength training and gained weight. That doesn't surprise me. It is one reason why I caution clients about putting too much stock in the bathroom scale. Pound for pound, muscle takes up about five times less space than fat.

Let's pretend I had 20 pounds of golf balls and 20 pounds of tennis balls. Then I poured each, respectively, into the legs of a pair of blue jeans. Which leg would be more full?

Of course, the leg with the tennis balls would be stuffed even though it weighed the same as the leg with the golf balls. In this case does it matter what the scale says? If you fit into a size six but weigh the same as you did when you wore a size 10 or 12, what difference does the scale make?

When embarking on a strength training program there is a transition period which can make some people uncomfortable. Muscle generally grows faster than fat shrinks. I wish it wasn't so. The results you get from a metabolic jump are slow and steady, where as hypertrophy, or muscle enlargement, happens relatively quickly.

There is quite a debate among fitness professionals about the amount of calories burned by a pound of muscle. However, two separate university studies, Tufts University[1] and The University of Maryland[2], found an increase of three pounds of muscle resulted in a 6.8% to 7.7% increase in the resting metabolism of the test subjects.

What does this mean to you? It could mean the loss of about one pound of fat monthly while at rest. Also, strength training burns additional calories for hours after your work-

---

[1] Campbell, W., Crim, M., Young, V., and Evans, W. "Increased energy requirements and changes in body composition with resistance training in older adults." *American Journal of Clinical Nutrition* 60: 167-175, 1994

[2] Pratley, R.., Nicklas, B., Rubin, M., Miller, J., Smith, A., Smith, M., Hurley, B. and Goldberg, A. "Strength training increases resting metabolic rate and norepinephrine levels in healthy 50- to 65-year-old men." *Journal of Applied Physiology* 76: 133-137, 1994.

out. Even though for a while you may actually feel bigger, please don't let this discourage you. The magic will happen if you keep it up.

There are many calculations and assessments that can be done to determine where a person falls on the weight continuum: BMI, body fat measurements, waist to hip circumference ratio, or just the scale, but most of us know how our clothes fit and where we would like to be.

Sometimes these measurements do more harm than good. Instead of seeking a change of life and health, we begin to gauge our success by a number. I've seen many people in bondage to their scales. Their mood for the day was determined when they stepped on their scale in the morning.

Strength training is good for more than just weight loss. It prevents the loss of lean body mass that happens from dieting and aging. It changes your lean to fat ratio, which helps shape your body and keep you healthy. It strengthens bones and connective tissue, which keeps you strong and active as you age. It improves coordination, balance, and helps prevent injuries.

As I said before, when one is attempting a lifestyle change, excess fat is lost much more slowly, but it's lost *permanently*. This program isn't an artificial diet. (How many times can I say it?) Therefore, you will not lose fat rapidly.

Our job is to train and transform ourselves from one kind of creature to another kind of creature. How much fat you lose in any given time frame depends on how long you have lived one way, how many changes you're willing and able to successfully implement, your body type, the amount of excess fat you're carrying, life's interruptions, and so on.

Meditate On It

Adding strength training to your workout schedule can be less painful than you think. You don't need to do a lot of it. Usually, 20 to 30 minutes two to three times a week can make a significant difference. Here are some tips for successful strength gains.

- Do exercises working all the major muscle groups. Muscles can get out of balance if you try to target only certain areas. We've all seen the muscle bound guy who's starting to look like King Kong because he is so focused on developing his chest, he has neglected the muscles of his back.
- During a workout, work your muscles from largest to smallest. It's best to begin with legs or chest and work your way down to the smaller muscles like biceps and shoulders. Save heavy abdominal work for last since your abdominal muscles support your back during the other exercises. You don't want to exhaust them on the front end.
- Get variety in your workout. Mix it up. It will help prevent boredom and injury. Try using your own body weight instead of free weights and do pushups, dips, or a TRX workout. Take a boot camp, Pilates, or an athletic Yoga class for a different kind of strength workout.
- Make sure you get sufficient rest. Your muscles hypertrophy, or grow stronger, when you're resting, not while you are lifting. Your body needs at least 48 hours between strength training sessions to recover.
- Continually challenge yourself. As you grow stronger the challenge should increase, or you will stop seeing strength gains.

Meditation

"Our real problem, then, is not our strength today; it is rather the vital necessity of action today to ensure our strength tomorrow."
- Dwight D. Eisenhower

Tip #8

Chocolate Helps Balance Your Blood Sugar

Chocolate in its natural state is a low glycemic food containing flavonoids that aid with insulin efficiency. Even with added cane sugar, dark chocolate in small amounts will have a beneficial effect on blood sugar regulation.

During the 1600's Catholics began drinking cocoa during fast days because it reduced hunger brought on by low blood sugar. This started a debate in Rome over whether chocolate should be allowed during religious fasts.

Adding raw cocoa to your smoothie in the morning may help you stick to your healthy eating goals throughout the day.

Nine

Having A Food Fight

I can't be young forever, but I want to look that way. I know I'm not alone in this because the plastic surgery business thrives even during economic downturns. For those of us who can't afford the high price tag, or are terrified of knives and needles, is there anything we can do to keep up appearances? Health and wellness experts say, "Yes."

Oxidation on a cellular level is apparently the primary cause of the sags, bags, dull skin tone, and dull wits occurring as we age. The fix is twofold. We must avoid the things promoting oxidation and do things to assist our body in fighting it.

So what do I have to avoid? Most doctors agree, while 20 to 30 minutes of sun a day is great for vitamin D production, over exposure to the sun will damage our skin and make us look old before our time. There is some controversy over sunblock, but I've never met a dermatologist who didn't say it was necessary to apply one every day. Try to find a sunblock with the most natural ingredients you can.

Some foods help our bodies fight the effects of the sun as

well. Tomatoes are high in lycopene, which has been shown to reduce the skin's sensitivity to sun, working like a natural sun block. Another perk is it increases collagen production. Collagen is what keeps our skin elastic.

There is also a growing body of research relating caffeine consumption with a reduction in the risk of skin cancer. Since coffee and tea are right up there on my list of never-say-no-to foods, this was good news for me. (I titled this book *The Wine and Chocolate Workout,* but I'm thinking of doing a sequel, *The Coffee and Green Tea Treatment.*)

Ingesting toxins is another way to age yourself quickly. That sounds like a silly statement. Who would knowingly eat poison? Most of us do it every day. Processed foods—things containing ingredients on the banned ingredient list from the *Kitchen Cleanse* exercise on page 44—would all fall into this category.

Over the counter medications and many prescription drugs are also very toxic to your system. It is estimated over 100,000 Americans die each year from taking their medications as directed. That number doesn't take into consideration all those who've suffered unusual adverse side effects, or fallen victim to the long term effects of drugs on the body. Unless it is absolutely essential to take a pill, other than supplements, I don't do it. Smoking and alcohol abuse are both, of course, very hard on your health.

Chronic stress is detrimental to your physiology on many levels. It promotes immune system deficiencies and early aging. The hormone cortisol is released in high-stress situations to assist your body in the fight or flight response to danger.

If you live with high levels of cortisol because of your job, relationships, or other environmental issues, it will have a damaging effect. It interrupts your sleep patterns, your body's ability to metabolize sugar, it increases abdominal fat, and it creates inflammation. Inflammation has many negative side effects, not the least of which is the breakdown of collagen in our skin leading to, ugh, wrinkles.

What can we do about stress? I get stressed out just thinking about it. Most of us aren't at liberty to quit our jobs, dump our spouse and wayward children, or move to a serene, pastoral village and start growing our own organic vegetables. Instead we must apply the three-pronged approach to making a life change.

Moderation:

Most of us think of moderation only as it pertains to potentially *fattening* substances, like wine and chocolate, but over-indulgence, even in good things, creates stress in our bodies. Moderation is another way of saying balance, and finding the balance in all things—exercise, eating, social and work habits—has a calming effect on our lives. The feeling of being out of control, while it may be exciting at times, is stressful. Overindulgence, while it might be fun on a special occasion, will create chronic stress if it becomes a lifestyle.

Meditation:

How you process life, what you focus on, is a source of great strength or great stress. Rick Warren, author of *The Purpose Driven Life,* says he used to think of life as a series of ups and downs, hills and valleys. Sometimes life was good, and other times it was difficult.

He has a different perspective now. He looks at life as a railroad track. There are two rails, one represents the blessings in life and the other the difficulties. They run parallel to each other, and it takes both to get you where you want to go. When we focus only on the difficulties, or the fun, we tend to get derailed.

Acceleration:

Exercise is crucial to controlling the stress in your life. Cardiovascular workouts produce endorphins which elevate your mood. I have had a number of clients who were able to stop taking antidepressant medications once they established a regular exercise routine.

Exercise gives an outlet to the adrenaline and cortisol released by stress. Remember these are the fight or flight hormones—so fly and fight. Go for a run or take a kickboxing class, and you've completed the cycle. The energy expenditure will also help you sleep at night, and sleep is an essential part of stress control.

Nutritional Stress Fighters

Finally, there are many foods high in anti-oxidative micronutrients. They can help our bodies fight the effects of toxins and stress we can't avoid.

It is better to attempt to fend off disease and early aging with nutrition rather than drugs. Drugs should be a last resort. Here are just a few, fabulous super foods:

- **Berries** - Blueberries, blackberries, black and red grapes, and blackcurrants contain phytochemicals which are powerful antioxidants. Red grapes are also high in resveratrol which is purported to prolong life. Wine tasting is good for your mood and your health.
- **Garlic** - Garlic helps to reduce cholesterol if eaten daily. It actually works better than aspirin to keep your blood thin, and this lowers your risk of heart disease. It also helps protect your body from cancer.
- **Green Vegetables** - All green vegetables, including

leafy greens, broccoli, Brussels sprouts, and lettuce, help fight toxins and fill you up with a very low calorie cost.

- **Avocado** - Avocados assist the body in lowering levels of bad cholesterol and are a great source of vitamin E, which promotes healthy, younger looking skin. Avocados may also help prevent hot flashes for those in that phase of life.
- **Nuts** - Almost all nuts are high in the minerals we need for our digestive and immune systems, but they are also high in calories. A little goes a long way. A serving of almonds is about 22 to 24 nuts.
- **Watermelon** - Contrary to the popular myth that you shouldn't eat watermelon seeds, when eaten they actually help, along with the fruit itself, to protect your body from free radicals. Free radicals can cause premature aging among other things. Juicing may help the seeds go down a little easier.
- **Whole Grains** - Whole grains are rich in minerals, fiber, and vitamins. They lower your risk of cardiovascular disease, cancer, and premature aging. However, more and more people are developing an intolerance to gluten which is in wheat, rye, barley, and some oats. There are several informative websites on this topic. If you have any of the symptoms, I suggest talking to your doctor about being tested for Celiac disease.
- **Teas** - Green and white teas are very high in antioxidants which help reduce the risk of some cancers, heart disease, and wrinkles. They are also thermogenic herbs which boost your metabolism, making it easier to lose weight.
- **Olive, Grape Seed, Flax Seed, and Coconut Oils** - Healthy oils are anti-inflammatory and help reduce

the incidence of age-related diseases like cancer, cardiovascular disease, and arthritis.

- **Fish** - Fish is rich in omega-3 fatty acids which is great for our brain, helps improve muscle tone, and prevents certain cancers. Caution: farm raised fish doesn't have the same benefits as wild caught and some studies show it may actually be harmful to your health.
- **Dark Chocolate** - I saved the best for last. Dark chocolate is extremely high in flavonoids which, when consumed on a daily basis, make skin softer, smoother, and better hydrated. They also appear to increase brain function so you can remember how to put your make up on.

Meditation

"*Wrinkled was not one of the things I wanted to be when I grew up.*" - Author Unknown

Tip #9

Chocolate Can Make You Look Younger

The antioxidants in dark chocolate help combat a number of aging enemies: sun, pollution, and anxiety, to name a few. Environmental and internal stresses cause inflammation in your body. Inflammation causes a world of damage, including a breakdown of collagen, and collagen breakdown causes wrinkles.

Dark chocolate not only cools inflammation and supports collagen repair, its healthy fats improve skin hydration, and the tryptophan in chocolate will ease your stress

You have completed Mesocycle Three

Take a week off to make these adjustments permanent. Rest a little in your workouts, and prepare for the final phase of the journey.

WINE WILL MAKE YOU MORE ATTRACTIVE

"Beer is made by men, wine by God." - Martin Luther

Wine is lovely. The range of translucent colors it yields and the countryside where it is produced are both visually stunning. We appreciate the beauty of wine, but can wine make us more beautiful?

The health benefits of wine are widely touted. It can help prevent heart disease, obesity, certain cancers, dementia, and many of the effects of aging. Since none of these conditions are particularly attractive, it's safe to say drinking wine in moderation will have a positive effect on our appearance.

Another obvious result of drinking wine is the influence it has on our mood. Wine has a euphoric effect. Studies have been done in which subjects were shown pictures of both smiling and neutral faces. The smiling faces won the beauty contest. People who appear cheerful are more attractive; wine makes you more cheerful, ergo wine makes you more attractive.

There are lesser known beautifying effects of wine, however. Apparently wine is good for your skin. The loss of collagen as we age is the primary cause of wrinkles. The polyphenols in wine help to maintain the skin's elasticity by promoting collagen production.

Wine also protects the skin from the UV rays of the sun, working as a kind of internal sun block. Sun damage is one of the leading causes of wrinkles and skin cancers. According to Dr. Oz, people who regularly drink wine tend to have a lower incidence of skin cancer.

The advantages of drinking wine for the skin are so pronounced, it has led some in the aesthetics field to dabble with the idea of using it topically. New wine based lotions, potions, and treatments are appearing on the market. A Spanish cosmetics company, with the help of a German chemical company, has developed a red wine powder which is added to skin creams to aid in the fight against wrinkles.

In France, the very first wine spa has opened its doors. They offer beauty treatments called vinotherapy. The claim is wine massages, wraps, and baths improve skin tone, reduce wrinkles, diminish cellulite, and provide temporary facelifts.

I don't know how I feel about using that much wine for purposes other than drinking. But if it works, what price for beauty? I do know this, after a glass or two of wine, I always think I look hotter. Maybe bathing in it would work wonders.

If you're feeling a little too frugal to try a hot tub full of vino, but you'd like to see if wine makes a difference on your skin, here's a recipe for a facial you can make at home.

Ingredients

1/3 cup yogurt
1/2 to 1 tbsp honey
2 to 3 tbsp red wine

Directions

Stir the wine, honey and yogurt until well blended. Massage mixture liberally onto a clean face. (It's okay to lick your fingers when you're done.) Leave on until the ingredients melt into the skin. Have a glass of wine and a piece of dark chocolate while you're waiting—just to belt and suspender the process. Rinse thoroughly.

MESOCYCLE FOUR

Finishing The Race

Your goal for this last mesocycle is to take all you've learned, make it your own, and run with it. Healthy living is an ever-growing, ever-changing process. You are making constant adjustments as situations alter your plans.

One of the biggest problems with diets and cookie-cutter programs is they make no room for the intrusions of life. What happens when you are injured and can't do the video workout? What happens when you have a week-long business trip and don't have access to the frozen food packets in your freezer? What happens when a family member has a crisis, and you are thrown into fear and depression? You stop your program and go back to what you've always done, which is exactly what got you into trouble in the first place.

The Wine and Chocolate Workout is for life. Habits remain habits even when life intrudes. If you've become a cardio junkie, and you sprain your ankle, you find a pool and swim for a couple of months. If you're acclimated to healthy eating and have to go out of town, you find a local health food store and chose wisely in restaurants. If a family member has a crisis, you know going for a long run or walk will give you time to work out issues and come back to the problem with more wisdom. In other words, this new lifestyle has become YOURS. It's what you do when life is good, when it's bad, and when it's neutral.

Meditation Exercise - Know Yourself

If you are like most people, you have gone on many diets and exercise programs over the years. Think back to those times. What did you try to accomplish and what knocked you off course?

____

____

____

____

Journal Work:

In column one below, list all the prior attempts you've made to lose weight and get in shape. In column two, write what actually happened and why.

Attempt	Result

Do you see a pattern?

____

____

____

____

What can you learn about yourself from this pattern?

____

____

____

____

How can you stop it?

____

____

____

____

Knowing yourself is key to making permanent lifestyle changes. Chapter ten will give you some strategies to assist with the above.

Moderation Exercise - Fight Back

After reading about the wonderful anti-oxidative properties in many foods in the last chapter, don't you feel like adding some to your diet? I love it when I'm supposed to eat something, instead of constantly being told what I can't eat. Most of my clients don't eat all the things they should. They say it is too time consuming. The answer to that is planning.

Journal Work:

Take out your meal plans and grocery lists and add a few of the foods mentioned in the chapter on *Having a Food Fight* each week this mesocycle. Find fun ways to prepare them, and make them a part of your regular diet.

Which foods am I going to add?

____

____

____

When am I going to add them?

____

____

____

How am I going to prepare them?

____

____

____

Acceleration Exercise - Grow Strong

You're becoming a regular fitness guru. You now know more about exercise than your average athlete, who usually only knows their sport. It's time to add one more discipline to your workout life—strength training.

Start slowly in this area. You really only need to do about 20 minutes of strength training twice a week. Just follow the guidelines in the *Being Leaner and Meaner* chapter, and throw a few heavy objects around this month. But, don't forget your cardio and core training.

Journal Work:

Add some strength training into your exercise schedule. Where, when, what, and how much? Be specific when you plan.

Sunday	Monday	Tuesday	Wednesday	Thursday	Friday	Saturday

TEN
Playing The Game

I know a woman who works with brain trauma patients. She was telling me about some of the crazy things the patients say to the nurses. She explained, the part of the brain acting as a filter between their thoughts and their mouths is often damaged. So brain trauma patients say whatever pops into their heads without thinking. I immediately asked (without thinking) if it was possible to be born without this filter?

I have had to learn this truth: Just because it is in my mind, doesn't mean it has to come out of my mouth. This is probably obvious to many of you. For me, not so much.

Here are some things I've learned are better left unsaid: How one can modify an exercise for pregnancy before you are sure the woman you're working with is, in fact, pregnant. Calling the tail of a turkey a "popesnose" at very Catholic, new mother-in-law's house, because you never realized "popesnose" is not an avian, anatomical term but is actually "Pope's nose." And, telling all my life altering plans, hopes, and dreams to someone who is unhappy with their current condition and has no intention of changing.

I have learned, the hard way, people who are wallowing in the mud of their own making don't like to see others get cleaned up and leave the sty. They will do whatever they can to pull you back into the muck. They will offer you all kinds of tempting slop and tell you about the horrifying slaughterhouses out there. Even those you thought were friends will sling mud at you as you leave. Save your pearls of wisdom for others who are on their own climb up and out. However, having said all that, there is always family.

Family sabotage is a huge problem for some people. Frequently I hear: "My husband won't eat vegetables." "My kids are so picky, about all they'll eat is hot dogs and pizza." "My family gets irritated when I take time out for exercise." "Every time I start an exercise program, one of my kids gets sick, and then I'm stuck in the house."

If this sounds familiar, don't despair. Almost any problem can be overcome if you can predict it and plan for it. You have two goals here: The first is to keep yourself on track and not allow the naysayers to derail you. The second is to evangelize your family.

The farther along you get in *The Wine and Chocolate Workout* lifestyle, the better you will feel, and the more benefits you'll see. When the transformation happens, you'll want to share everything you've learned with those you love. However, often they won't listen. The Bible says a prophet is least respected in his own hometown.

Note to Parents

Your kids will be healthier and happier if they have healthier, happier parents. Martyrs may be admirable, but they are no fun to live with. Sacrificing everything for your children isn't good for either them or you. Keep that in mind when you're torn between getting in your workout or driving the kids to one more activity.

The statistics on childhood obesity and the accompanying illnesses are very scary. Even if your children are thin, the habits you model for them now will probably stay with them for their lifetime. It's likely those patterns will also affect how they will raise *their* children.

Offensive Strategies

If you don't have children, you still probably have a significant other or extended family whose health you care about. Developing both offensive and defensive strategies with your family is essential at some point in the lifestyle change process, or you will fall back into old habits and never alter theirs. I happen to believe the best defense is a good offense.

An offensive strategy shouldn't actually be offensive, if you catch my drift. They say there is nothing worse than a reformed prostitute, or alcoholic, or smoker, or—fill in the blank. You need to resist the desire to preach at your family, or act holier-than-thou. Nobody likes to be manipulated, or forced into things.

Instead, apply the training principles from chapter one to your family, but don't tell them you're doing it. Well, maybe tell your spouse, but not your kids. Being a little sneaky can go a long way toward improving your family's health.

Training means making small changes with consistency and allowing yourself to physically and mentally adapt before another change is introduced.

When it comes to your family, begin to introduce new ideas, foods, and exercise opportunities into their lives in small consistent steps. Instead of sending the kids to school with chips in their lunch bags, put in flavored rice or soy cakes. Let them keep the white bread for another month, then one day try a mixed whole and white wheat bread. A few weeks later switch to 100% whole grain bread.

Some week suggest Frisbee in the park before the Friday night video. Do it several weeks in a row, and it will become a tradition. Don't try to change their entire lives in one week, or even in one month. Do things little by little.

Give them pizza or fast food, but cut down on the frequency. Instead of McDonald's, Little Caesars, and Taco Bell all in one week, how about only one fast food stop and make great healthy tacos, burgers, and pizza at home more often?

Training will actually alter the physical makeup of your body, change your emotional state, and give you knowledge you can't unlearn.

As you gradually change the family menu and the kinds of foods you have in the house, their bodies will adapt. They will learn to enjoy those foods. Don't let the grousing deter you, and don't tell them you're trying to change them. Present healthy meals, and act enthusiastic about them yourself.

It's good to educate others in a non-challenging way as you learn. It is said, the best way to get something deeply ingrained in your own soul is to share it with someone else. Share what you learn about the benefits of cardiovascular exercise while you're out playing with your kids or walking the dog with your mate. Your family will gain knowledge they can't unlearn, while you reinforce it within yourself.

I read an article about what happens in your body when you eat a doughnut. It was very distressing. I shared what I learned with my husband—a confirmed doughnut hound. He, subsequently, cut doughnuts back from a weekly habit to an occasional extravagance. I didn't lecture. I educated.

Training disciplines your body, working with it to bring out your natural strengths and abilities; it is not about punishment.

My grandmother always said you catch more flies with honey than with vinegar. Encouragement and sincere compliments work much better than nagging. I don’t know about you, but I need to post that on my wall and read it every day.

Look for ways to accentuate your family’s natural strengths and abilities. Many people's children are in sports, so they think the exercise thing is handled. Unless those kids are talented and driven enough to be professional athletes, they often fall off the exercise wagon in adulthood. Most adults don't participate in team sports. If that is their only experience with exercise, they're at risk.

I taught a year-long class for high school juniors and seniors called *Fitness for Life*. In that class we explored the world of adult fitness. They got credit for any type of exercise they did. As a result, they tried all kinds of gym classes, weight lifting, skiing, surfing, and even triathlon training.

Help your family find their strengths, just as you had to do when you first started this process. If your kids run really well in soccer, try running with them in the off-season, or maybe running a 5K together. If they swim well, take some family water vacations where they can enjoy their ability without whistles, time goals, and bathing caps.

My husband and daughter mountain bike together. Not only is it great exercise for both of them, it is a bonding time as well. My daughter is also extremely flexible. I have gone to Yoga and hip hop with her. On family vacations, we all hike together.

When basketball began to cause too many injuries in my husband's life, I talked him into running with me. He had been the captain of the track team in high school. I knew that talent was buried in there somewhere. He now runs circles around me. We plan and train for races together, even though he gets to the finish line way ahead of me.

Defensive Strategies

In regards to making a lifestyle change, I think a good defense is essential too. What I mean is, setting an example is worth 1,000 words, or more. If your family sees you changing and growing in your health and fitness, it will speak volumes to them.

Studies have shown children of alcoholics are more likely to abuse alcohol. Children of smokers are more likely to smoke. Children of overweight parents are more likely to be overweight. And, children of exercising parents are more likely to have an active lifestyle. This is great motivation to keep you going when you want to quit.

However, if you have already set one family pattern into motion and now you're rocking the boat, it is very likely there will be some complaining. The only thing I can say to this is, keep moving forward quietly. If you have a headache, you take a pain killer. If you have a pain in the neck in your house, here are some painkillers you can take:

- Call one of your cheerleaders for a pep-talk
- Read a motivational book
- Watch athletes on T.V. and get inspired
- Go for a walk, run, swim, or some kind of workout
- Review your progress, and appreciate yourself for how far you've come
- Pray

If your situation is really destructive, I highly recommend marriage and family counseling. I once had a client who was about 125 pounds overweight. When she married she was a healthy weight and an avid runner. But, hubby was a feeder. In 10 years of marriage, she doubled in size.

She was working out with me several days a week and was making great headway in her eating habits, when her husband started to sabotage her. He brought home large meat-lovers pizzas, two-pound boxes of chocolates, and all kinds of fast-foods. He said he was rewarding her for her efforts.

It was obvious this weight loss stuff was making him nervous. Not knowing what else to do, she began taking his food gifts straight to the trash. He finally admitted he was afraid she would leave him if she got fit. This was out of my league. They needed professional counseling.

I had another client who had the opposite issue. Her husband was constantly monitoring her every bite. At a party, she decided to have a small brownie. This was a conscious decision with her daily calorie allotment taken into consideration. Her husband saw her and immediately commented, "Are you sure you should be eating that?"

She was so humiliated and angry, she ate five brownies just to spite him. This event opened her eyes. The person she hurt was herself. She needed to stop allowing him to influence her negatively.

We don't live in a vacuum. The reason we are the way we are, the reason we pick the significant others we pick, the reason our children have the habits they have, is because of relationships, past and present. Some are healthy. Some aren't.

If you want to change a lifetime of habits, you will have to spend time evaluating your relationships. You may need to alter situations that are harmful to your health. Blaming others, or allowing them to have undue influence on you, is not productive. If you need help, get help, but don't throw up your hands and give in or give up.

Meditate on it

Mealtimes are often the most dangerous times in families. As you're working on implementing change in your household, realize you don't have to eat everything you cook for them, or they cook for you. You can make other things for yourself. I take a little bit of the meat, or whatever the main dish is, and beef it up with vegetables. Turn tacos into taco salad, or spaghetti into pasta primavera. I often make spaghetti squash for myself and regular pasta for the family.

Think up healthy desserts you enjoy, and have them when everyone else is eating ice cream. Baked apples with cinnamon and Greek yogurt is as good as apple pie in my book.

Journal Work:

Write down three typical family meals, include desert if you normally have it. Use this space to brainstorm how you could modify them to make them more *Wine and Chocolate Workout* friendly.

Meal #1

____

____

____

____

Meal #2

____

____

____

____

Meal #3

____

____

____

____

Meditation

"The task of a leader is to get his people from where they are to where they have not been." - Henry Kissinger

Tip #10

Chocolate is Good for Your Sex Life (I Think)

Chocolate has been considered an aphrodisiac since the days of the ancient Aztecs. There is some science to back this up. The chemical phenylethylamine is present in high levels when a person is aroused and drops to the basement when love is unrequited. Chocolate does contain phenylethylamine, but scientists say it's not present in high enough quantities to actually make a difference.

I wouldn't minimize the placebo effect however. I, for one, think chocolate is sexy. If you don't agree, make sure you try Tip #11

ELEVEN
Amping It Up

There is a very interesting mathematical principle which states 20 percent of output is responsible for 80 percent of input. In other words, 20 percent of your efforts are responsible for 80 percent of your results. This tends to be true in economics, business, and just about every area of life.

I've seen many runners who run mile after mile, year after year, in long distance races but never get any faster. Not only do they not get faster, but often they don't lose any additional weight once the novelty of running has worn off on their body. I've also seen people who take indoor cycling classes three to five times a week for years who, likewise, never show any dramatic signs of improvement after the initial adaptation period. They are spending 80 percent of their time for a 20 percent advantage.

Training means making small changes with consistency and allowing yourself to physically and mentally adapt before another change is introduced

These people made a change, and their bodies adapted. Then they stopped training, and the progress stopped. Don't let this statement overwhelm you. You don't have to invest more time to exercise, just exercise smarter.

Apply the 80/20 principle. Don't increase your time commitment; instead, figure out the most effective 20 percent of what you are doing and do more of that and less of the 80 percent which is not as effective.

In the case of exercise, change is effective. Do something different. "But I like my sport," you say. This is where interval training comes in.

Interval Training

Interval training is a workout designed to raise your fitness level by incorporating short bursts of high intensity exercise into a routine. There are many benefits to interval training for both the seasoned athlete and for the beginner.

Most people have been told long-duration, low-intensity exercise—such as a moderate-paced walk—burns more fat than a shorter high-intensity workout. This is only true in a proportional sense. You burn a higher percentage of fat as your primary fuel when doing lower level cardiovascular work, but you burn so much more fuel at higher intensities, you ultimately burn more fat. Here are some of the advantages to adding interval training into your workout:

- It trains your body to handle higher intensities more quickly
- It boosts your metabolism for an extended period, even after the workout is completed
- It enables you to burn more fuel in a shorter period of time
- You achieve many of the physical benefits of working at a high intensity for a longer time

- It builds confidence in your ability to handle higher levels of exercise, so you are more likely to advance
- It relieves boredom
- It's an easy way to measure your performance
- You see improvement quickly, which is very motivating

There are many ways to add interval training into your workouts. For example, if you want to turn your walks into runs, alternate walking four minutes and running one, for two miles. Over time increase your running to two minutes, three minutes and so on; this will prepare your body for running longer periods.

Once you are able to run for 2 miles, you can begin to increase your speed the same way. Run a short distance—say 200 meters—at a faster pace than you normally would, slow back to your jog, then repeat. Over time increase to 400 meters, 800 meters, a half mile and so on. You will establish a much quicker pace for distance runs.

If you don't want to run, you can add intensity to your walks with hill climbs. A couple of days a week pick a difficult course with steep hills. The second week, walk up and down the hills two or three times each time you come to one. You can shorten the course on your hill climb days. Just find some big hills to repeat in increasing numbers and with increasing speed.

Circuit training can become interval training if it is approached correctly. In a circuit training workout, you move from exercise to exercise based on timing or number of repetitions. If cardiovascular exercise is interspersed with strength work, an interval effect can be achieved.

For instance, if you did ten pushups, ten pull ups, ten lunges, and ten squats with 3 minutes of jump rope in between each set, you would be working at varying cardiovascular intensities. This would achieve the same effect on your heart as hill climbs or running sprints, and you'd be getting strength training at the same time.

Boot camp, circuit, and indoor cycling classes are a good place to experience interval training. Sports such as basketball and tennis, in which you run full speed for short distances, have an interval training effect as well.

But remember, even classes and sports that are interval oriented can become blasé to your body. If you are doing those kinds of activities regularly, you might need to do some longer duration, steady-state training to shake things up. The point is, as soon as something becomes easy and comfortable, you need to amp it up and make a change of some kind.

A note of warning, interval training can be very intense. Make sure you pace yourself. You should be able to repeat your most intense interval at least three times with a minute or two of rest in between. If you can't, you're working at too high a threshold. Also, injuries can occur at high levels if you're not properly warmed up. Warm up for at least ten minutes at moderate intensity before your workout, and treat yourself to a ten minute cool down afterwords.

Meditate On It

Three months is long enough to get into a rut. Are you ready for a challenge? It's time to shake up your exercise life yet again.

Journal Work:

What kind of cardiovascular exercise you are currently doing?

____

____

____

How could you turn this sport or activity into an interval training?

___

___

___

How could you save time by incorporating strength training exercises with cardiovascular exercise?

___

___

___

What are two other kinds of interval training workouts you might like to try?

___

___

___

Meditation

"We can't become what we need to be by remaining who we are." - Richard V. Howard

Tip #11

Have a Chocolate Massage

With all the health benefits gained by eating chocolate, it's no wonder somebody got the bright idea to rub it all over themselves. Many micro-nutrients are absorbed quickly through the skin and the oil in chocolate is very moisturizing. Chocolate massages are in vogue in spas around the world.

If you'd like a more personal and less expensive chocolate massage experience, here is a recipe for Chocolate Body Lotion.

Ingredients:

1 ounce cocoa butter
1/2 ounce almond or grape seed oil
Chocolate scented essential oil.

Directions:

Place the cocoa butter in the top of a double boiler. Heat until completely melted. Whisk in almond or grape seed oil until it's a good consistency. You can add more oil if you like thinner lotion. Add 3 or 4 drops of chocolate essential oil, or more if you want a stronger scent. Pour into a clean, glass container. Cover tightly. Have fun.

TWELVE
Crossing The Finish Line

For the past 12 weeks, you've been led through a series of weekly tweaks. Hopefully, some of these changes have become habits you no longer have to think about. You may be tempted to close the book and pat yourself on the back. You've arrived.

I hate to be the bearer of bad news, *but there's really no such thing as maintenance*. Stagnation breeds algae. You're either progressing, or going backwards. It's time to own your new lifestyle. I'd like to leave you with a few thoughts and tools for continuing on along the *Wine and Chocolate Workout* path.

At one point I was going to call my blog *The Weekly Tweak.* My children laughed out loud when they heard the title. "Of course you'd be thin if you were tweaking, Mom. Who needs a blog about that?" Apparently, tweaking is a term used for doing methamphetamine. Thank you, kids. However, I still like the concept.

Weekly Tweaks

A weekly tweak, in my book, is the process of taking some time on a regular basis to evaluate your progress. To examine what's working for you, what's not, and make small changes. To reiterate the 80/20 Rule from the last chapter, 20 percent of output is responsible for 80 percent of input. It's very important to pause and attempt to decipher which 20 percent leads to the greatest success.

Entrepreneurial Mindset Check-ups

Another tool is the entrepreneurial mindset check-up. In the first mesocycle we learned we need to be *entrepreneurial eaters*. I want to expand on that concept. I believe we need to have an entrepreneurial mindset in all areas of life. Remember Webster's definition of an entrepreneur is: *one who organizes, manages and assumes the risk of an enterprise.*

Take a little quiz. Are you now more entrepreneurial than you were 12 weeks ago? Use this list every so often to make sure you haven't fallen back into old, bad habits.

Entrepreneurial Eater

- You are constantly evolving
- You see eating habits as unique to each individual
- You accept personal responsibility
- You are thoughtful and involved
- You take the best from many sources
- Health is your measure of success
- Your reward is nourishment and enjoyment
- You are motivated by a positive self-image
- You accept and work with reality

Defeatist Dieter

- You follow a stagnant, predetermined set of rules
- You follow a one-size-fits-all plan
- You blame or praise the diet for failure or success
- You are mindlessly obedient
- You rely on one source
- The scale is your measure of success
- Your punishment is deprivation and guilt
- You are motivated by a poor body image
- You often foster unrealistic expectations

Drawing Lines in the Sand

Besides weekly tweaks and entrepreneurial mindset check-ups, I believe in drawing lines in the sand. A line in the sand is a predetermined place where, once arrived at, an action or decision must occur. Where you draw your line may be different than where I draw mine, but we all need to have the same response when we come up against it—make a change.

For me, the line is my jeans. When my jeans start getting too tight, it's time to pull out my iPhone and start charting calories in and calories out to see where I'm going astray.

For you, it might be a number on the scale, a fitness test (how fast you can run a certain distance, or how many pushups you can do), a blood pressure or cholesterol number, or how many headaches you're getting a week. Decide in advance what you're not willing to put up with. Decide what you're going to do about it when the line is crossed.

Continuing Education

Consider yourself a lifelong student of wellness. Hopefully, you'll be living in your body for a long time to come.

Maintaining it is one of the most important things you can do. You will think better, feel better, have more energy and therefore be more successful at whatever you set your hand to if you're living healthfully. Make it a habit to learn something new regularly. whether it's a new exercise format, a new recipe, or the latest research on coconuts.

The point of this process is to find your own permanent path to success, a plan uniquely tailored to your life, body, likes and dislikes. Often this will come in stages. The steps you were willing to make in the first mesocycle may be very different than those you're willing to take today.

As you progress in fitness, you will find yourself accomplishing things you couldn't imagine yourself doing in the past. I guarantee, if you stay on the *Wine and Chocolate Workout* path, the changes in your life will be radical in a year, two years, and five years down the road.

Meditation

"Twenty years from now you will be more disappointed by the things you didn't do than by the one you did do. So throw off the bowlines. Sail away from the safe harbor. Catch the trade winds in your sails. Explore. Dream. Discover." - Mark Twain

TIP #12

Chocolate, the Secret Ingredient

In the 1500's, British pirates captured a Spanish ship filled with a precious cargo, cocoa beans. Chocolate was such a well kept Spanish secret at the time, the pirates had no idea what it was. They thought the dark seeds were sheep droppings and burned them all.

The moral of the story is: Share the secrets of wine and chocolate.

Wine and Chocolate Will Make You a Better Person

"Men are like wine–some turn to vinegar, but the best improve with age." - Pope John XXIII

As you are now aware, self-discipline is an essential ingredient in a healthy lifestyle. However, too much is just obnoxious. Wine and chocolate can be your saving graces.

There is a character on the T.V. show *Parks and Rec* named Chris Traeger. He is a health fanatic. He runs 10 miles a day, is a vegetarian, takes endless supplements, is unwaveringly positive, and generally insufferable. I cringe a little when I watch him. I don't want to be a stereotypical fitness nut, and I definitely have more things in common with him than I do most of the other characters on the show.

We don't want to be like the Chris Traeger's of the world. This is why it is so important to indulge in wine and chocolate. I know, you will argue wine and chocolate are actually good for you in moderation. So how much of an indulgence are they? Well, sometimes I think we should throw moderation out the window, how's that?

Don't get me wrong, we need to exercise restraint, but at the same time, we need to guard against becoming self-righteous prigs. To most people's thinking, I'm am a very self-disciplined person. I eat lots of fresh veggies, work out, drink water, take my supplements, avoid sugar and other simple carbs, eat gluten free, and feel whole grain brown rice crackers with organic peanut butter are a splurge. But, I let myself eat, drink, and be merry at least once a week. Why? Because I've seen people turn this healthy lifestyle thing into a religion.

What are the signs you've turned into a fitness fanatic?

- You begin to feel and act superior to other people
- You're no fun to be around, because you make other people feel bad about themselves
- You become self-absorbed and selfish about your habits
- You begin to restrict where you'll go and who you'll spend time with based on how healthy the occasion will be
- You become competitive with others who exercise and try to eat right

Not only will you be very lonely, because no one will like you, but one day you'll probably blow up and eat an entire package of bacon topped with chocolate cake and ice cream.

Personally, I think it is much better to let yourself enjoy life a little. You will have a better perspective, more friends, and return to your health goals refreshed. God made wine to make the heart glad (Ps 104:14-15). I'm sure He had the same thing in mind when He created chocolate.

STAY IN TOUCH...

Congratulations. You have completed Mesocycle 4. Make sure you stay in touch with your biggest cheerleader–me.

Want more pearls of wisdom? Come visit me at gretaboris.com where I share brilliant thoughts about defeating our personal demons, stories of people who inspire me, and news about my writing life.

I'd love to hear about your wine and chocolate adventures. Let's be friends on social media. You can find me on Facebook: www.facebook.com/greta.boris and Twitter: @gretaboris

Stop by Gretaboris.com and download free work pages for The Wine and Chocolate Workout.

Resources

Wine Resources:

The Reverse Wine Snob - Thumbing my nose at bottles over $20

For those of you just getting into the wonderful world of wine, I love this website. Jon Thorsen and his wife decided to start drinking more wine due to all the lovely health benefits. This can get pretty pricey however. So they set out on a quest to find the best wines for under $20 a bottle. This site has a wealth of information, including reviews on Costco and Trader Jo wines. I check with Jon before I go shopping.

www.reversewinesnob.com

The Wine Wankers

A fun blog from down under that attempts to avoid the snobbery some wine writers and drinkers exude like the nose on a turned bottle. Follow the wine adventures of Ben, Neal, and Conrad as they drink around the globe.

www.thewinewankers.com.au

Cellar Angels

If you've read any of my wine articles, you know Cellar Angels are special friends. They not only represent some of the finest Napa Valley wineries and offer terrific prices for artisan wines, they give a percentage of all bottles sold to charity. And, Martin Cody and the gang are just nice folks. If you plan on joining a wine club, check them out.

www.cellarangels.com

Hoot n Annie - Drinking Wine for the People

Matt and Annie blog about the wine lifestyle on the Central Coast of California. Since this is one of my favorite places in the world, I'm a big fan. If you live on the West Coast or are planning a visit, Paso Robles and surrounds should be part of your travel agenda. I fantasize about moving to a small vineyard in San Luis Obispo.

www.www.hootnannieblog.com

Wine Match - Matching Wines You Like!

Have you ever tasted a wine you loved, then looked at the price and decided you didn't love it that much? Or, have you ever bought an expensive bottle on a recommendation, only to discover you didn't really care for it? Wine Match has a nifty tool to help you dial in your wine taste. You can locate wines you will like by finding comparisons to those you've enjoyed in the past.

www.winematch.com

Delectable

Delectable is a phone app that instantly recognizes any wine from its label. You can use it as a diary by simply taking a picture of the wine label and making notes. You can also search wines and instantly see others' reviews. If you're the social sort, you can make your list public, and see what your friends are drinking. Delectable will even help you track down a hard to find wine, so

you can order it direct. I wish I had this app years ago—so many lost loves, sigh.
www.delectable.com

Chocolate Resources:

The Santa Barbara Chocolate Company

No matter where you live, The Santa Barbara Chocolate Company is a fantastic resource for chocoholics looking for healthy, sustainable, organic chocolate. They offer everything from pure cacao chunks to lovely truffles.
www.santabarbarachocolate.com

Chocolate Therapy - Sweet Remedies

I've never been to this lovely shop, but next time I'm on the East Coast I'm going. I love their name, their perspective, and they do regular wine and chocolate tasting events. They have some really unique sweets, like blueberry lemon basil truffles (good with a pinot noir, I'm thinking) You can order custom chocolates from them, and yes, you can order online.
www.ctsweetremedies.com

Living Healthy with Chocolate

For those of you who prefer your chocolate mixed with more ingredients, this is a great recipe resource. Andriana Harlan has the right perspective when it comes to eating healthy. She tells her own story on this site. She offers lots of Paleo and gluten free recipes for those of you trying to cut back on the white stuff.
www.livinghealthywithchocolate.com

Got Chocolate - Celebrating All Things Chocolate

Laura Ruker is less focused on health and more on, well... chocolate. Anything and everything you ever wanted to know about chocolate, including some health facts and gluten free and diabetic recipes, will be found on Laura's site. This is a good place

for moms to drop by. She has some cute recipes for kids.
www.gotchocolate.com

Chocolate Covered Katie - The Healthy Dessert Blog

Katie's mission is to take all your favorite dessert recipes and make them healthier, especially if they contain chocolate. For instance, she has a new and improved version of a Reese's Peanut Butter Egg and gluten free cupcakes topped with her healthier Nutella.
www.chocolatecoveredkatie.com

General Weight Loss and Health Resources:

The Bikini Chef - Figure Flattering Flavors

A lot of people have told me I should have put recipes in this book, but I'm not much of a cook. Thank goodness there are some terrific chefs out there who share my foodie philosophy. Susan Irby is one. Susan has eight terrific cookbooks, a radio show all about the bikini lifestyle, and she's good people.
www.thebikinichef.com

Eat. Drink. Be Skinny.

Theresa Marie Howes is a bundle of healthy energy. She's the author of the original Skinnytinis—All the Fun for Half the Calories. (So, you know we're friends.) She has oodles of recipes, workout challenges, and a great new detox program on her blog.
www.eatdrinkandbeskinny.com

Elise Cohen Ho - Naturally Yours

Elise is a naturopathic health practitioner who has transformed her own life and body. Elise lost eighty pounds the right way and now teaches others. She has a wealth of encouraging, health-affirming information on her site, and you can actually work with her if you need a coach to help you navigate your life change.
www.elisecohenho.com

Dr. Mark Hyman

Dr. Mark Hyman is a leader in the field of functional medicine. He is the author of numbers of New York Times bestsellers including The Blood Sugar Solution. His website has loads of interesting and informative health articles you won't find in many other places.

www.drhyman.com

The Daniel Plan

If you're looking for a crowd to help you make this positive life change, check out The Daniel Plan. The Daniel Plan was started by Pastor Rick Warren (The Purpose Driven Life) in response to some health issues he was facing. It is a community driven program promoting Faith, Food, Fitness, Focus, and Friends as a path to success. Yours truly was involved in the early days. You can read an article I wrote for them here:

www.danielplan.com/healthyhabits/playbackintoexercise/

www.danielplan.com

CPSIA information can be obtained
at www.ICGtesting.com
Printed in the USA
LVOW04s1514120716
496010LV00038B/687/P

9 780692 323731